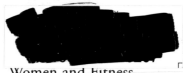

ALSO BY SARAH HENTGES

*Pictures of Girlhood: Modern Female
Adolescence on Film* (McFarland, 2006)

Women and Fitness in American Culture

SARAH HENTGES

McFarland & Company, Inc., Publishers
Jefferson, North Carolina, and London

LIBRARY OF CONGRESS CATALOGUING-IN-PUBLICATION DATA

Hentges, Sarah, 1976–
    Women and fitness in American culture / Sarah Hentges.
        p.   cm.
    Includes bibliographical references and index.

    ISBN 978-0-7864-7480-6
    softcover : acid free paper ∞

    1. Women—Health and hygiene—United States—
Sociological aspects.   2. Physical fitness for women—
United States—Social aspects.   3. Exercise for
women—United States—Social aspects.   I. Title.
    RA778.H457 2014
    613.7'045—dc23   2013038444

BRITISH LIBRARY CATALOGUING DATA ARE AVAILABLE

On the cover: woman in yoga pose with futuristic
interface (Wavebreak Media/Thinkstock)

Manufactured in the United States of America

*McFarland & Company, Inc., Publishers
    Box 611, Jefferson, North Carolina 28640
    www.mcfarlandpub.com*

Dedicated to all the women who love to lose themselves — and find themselves — through fitness.

"Like aerobicizing soldiers, the women move in unison, with a precision that even the military would admire. The bodies are obedient: to rhythm, to other participants, and to the directives of the instructor. But aerobics is being blamed for wider social traumas."
— Tara Brabazon, "Fitness Is a Feminist Issue"

"Now I walk in rhythmic patterns
Count beats to beat match the measures of
Old school pop with urban street hip-hop
And adjust my pulse accordingly"
— Shaden Tavakoli (Lady Sha),
"This DJ," *Home Girls Make Some Noise*

"We live in a culture that is 'body conscious,' and when women feel they have powerful bodies, they are empowered. Feeling empowered physically does wonders for one's mental and emotional well-being."
— Wendy Walter-Bailey, "If These Roads Could Talk:
Life as a Woman on the Run," *My Life at the Gym*

"Within the yoga studio, women can shuck the concretions of the mind and in that radical, momentary transformation form a powerful connection with each other. The intimacy of the studio's silence speaks its own language of community."
— Victoria Boynton, "Women's Yoga: A Multigenre Meditation
on Language and the Body," *My Life at the Gym*

"If I can't dance — I don't want to be part of your revolution."
— Emma Goldman (1869–1914)

Table of Contents

Acknowledgments

Moving in and around the worlds of fitness and academia for 15 years, teaching in Northern California, Oregon, Washington, Minnesota, and Maine, means that I have been inspired by far too many wonderful individuals to name here. Generally, I'd like to acknowledge all of my students and colleagues, and all of my supervisors, mentors, participants, and fellow instructors, who have supported, inspired, bolstered, and grounded me throughout my career. Some of you are mentioned in these pages; all of you are in my heart.

More immediately, many people were integral to helping me make this book a reality. Danielle Eastman and Amy Stroud both read my first full draft and gave me not only practical advice but also support and the confidence to keep working out the details. Lauren Verow helped with so many of the details, and she did so with patience and care. She also sent me some of the best fitness — and most feminist — related links that helped me deepen and expand my analysis. Several other people also sent fitting fitness sources my way: Erica Davis, Nick Bear, Michelle Moon, Sean Ames, Lisa Botshon, Ana Noriega and Tessa Hayes. Thank you to all of my students in AME/WST 304 in the fall of 2012 who read early drafts of some of this work and took up the subject matter of "American Fitness" with passion and a critical eye. You all produced excellent work, reflecting on personal and community and structural forms of fitness, making me realize the purpose and potential of this book. Special thanks to Kristin Dubay, Tessa Hayes, Kim Nixon, and Rillyria Sherifi who all continue to inspire me through their vision and passion. All of my students remind me, over and over, why I do the work I do.

Thank you to my Bangor YMCA fitness family and my University of Maine at Augusta colleagues, especially Lisa Botshon who helps me balance and Ellen Taylor who encouraged my "kinesthetic pedagogy." I'd also like to thank faculty members at the University of Maine who encouraged my early work on this project: Carla Billitteri, Mazie Hough, Renate Klein, and Ann Schonberger. Thanks also to Jo Malin and Tara Brabazon —first for their inspirational work, but mostly for their down-to-earth, approachable nature and enthusiastic support. It's always empowering when you realize your heroes are people too. And they return your emails.

Thanks to my family for their unconditional love and support. To my mountain goat who takes my fitness outside and to my mother who sparked my love of fitness, dance, and writing. After years of writing about your kids, I get to return the favor.

And finally, thanks to Tessa Pyles who has supported me through every variation of fitness dance I have created and explored, and who has travelled many miles — literally and figuratively — to dance with me, even when no one else would.

Preface

In American culture, trends rise and fall. I have tried to capture a moment — albeit an extended moment — in the history of American fitness. This is not a linear history; nor is it complete. It is a contemporary American history of fitness that challenges what the very terms of our inquiry mean. I sample diverse voices from across fitness cultures and contextualize these voices through my personal and professional experience. I try to do justice to these voices by letting them speak and by contextualizing them. I try to represent the trends, nuances, and layers of American fitness in all its complexity. My reach is expansive here and, yet, limited to a set of illustrative and representative examples. My bias is clear ... and foundational. I love "group fitness." And I see transformative potential in my academic work as well as my work out.

My work in American studies, women's studies, comparative ethnic studies, sociology, and cultural studies provides a set of lenses through which I consider popular culture and academic inquiries and forms a basis for the arguments put forth in this work. There are two important languages used throughout the book — the specialized terms of the fitness world and those of the world of academia. I do my best to balance and explain this language and its associated figures, approaches, and ideas. The term and concept of "fitness," however, is meant to be slippery and defined in context and complexity. Each part of *Women and Fitness in American Culture* develops and extends this concept — stretching, layering, transforming.

In an attempt to inspire readers to explore fitness in all of its dimensions, I use the full names of scholars and public figures; I also include endnotes for further explanations and a works cited section. These references, as well as the appendix of fitness terms, products, personalities, and brands and the index, can help connect the names, trends, and ideas that are layered throughout this book. I hope readers will draw their own conclusions and continue

1

this conversation in their own communities, universities, gyms, community centers, online spaces, and homes.

    I use first names only for my fitness friends and acquaintances; I expect they will recognize themselves here and I hope that they will see what I see. I hope that they will be inspired. I use anonymous descriptions for more personal revelations and explorations, and many of these examples apply to more than one particular individual. I hope that all readers will see themselves in these pages, and be inspired to move.

Introduction

"PHYSICAL FITNESS is not only one of the most important keys to a
healthy body, it is the basis of dynamic and creative intellectual activity. The relationship between the soundness of the body and the activities of the mind is subtle and complex. Much is not yet understood.
But we do know what the Greeks knew: That intelligence and skill can
only function at the peak of their capacity when the body is healthy
and strong; that hardy spirits and tough minds usually inhabit sound
bodies."

— President John F. Kennedy as quoted
by Kenneth Cooper in *Aerobics*

For more than four decades "fitness" has evolved in American culture
and consciousness. The publication of Dr. Kenneth Cooper's seminal work
in 1968 changed scientific and popular conceptions of fitness as either "freedom
from disease" or as the kind of peak conditioning of elite athletes, as Lt. General Richard L. Bohannon points out in his introduction to Cooper's *Aerobics*.
Since then, a variety of fitness forms have developed in the U.S. from early
incarnations of aerobics to interactive video game fitness programs, from Step
Aerobics to P90X, from boot camp to yoga. The cultural markers of Jane
Fonda and Wii Fit speak to a multifaceted evolution and frame my critical
and creative exploration of American mind/body fitness. One is a fitness personality, marketed to women, emulated in many incarnations and a symbol
of fitness in American consciousness, even when her politics have made her
unpopular; the other is a form of video game that interrupts the sedentary
and isolated lifestyle that such electronic conveniences (and our aversion to
exercise coupled with our poor eating habits) have helped shape among many
Americans. But these are only rough markers and instructive symbols. The
story of American fitness takes us from the White House to our living room,
from the individual pursuit to the collective interest, from manufactured to
creative art, within and beyond.

While Presidential standards of fitness have attempted to set the lead for American fitness over the past 45 years, the Obamas have entered the national conversation about health and fitness in a way that challenges Americans to rethink their relationship to their bodies and their food. Michelle Obama's Let's Move! initiative, coupled with organic gardening and healthy eating tips, has spread through media coverage of White House events as well as T.V. shows. Here we have the First Lady dancing on the White House lawn, adding a Yoga Garden to the annual Easter Egg Roll, working in the organic garden, visiting schools, doing push-ups with Ellen Degeneres, employing the help of pop culture, and working to change the way we think about our health and fitness. Greatist.com even named Michelle Obama as the number one most influential person in health and fitness in 2012. Encouraging movement reminds us just how stationary—literally and figuratively—Americans and America have become. And movement is both a fitness tool as well as a metaphor as we consider the state of fitness and the state of our nation.

Icons, technologies, and Presidential leadership are only part of the fitness story in America. Exploring American fitness through a critical lens reveals the ways in which we think about fitness as well as the ways in which this concept of fitness shapes our lives and culture. But more importantly, this exploration reveals how we can transform ourselves and our culture by rethinking what American fitness really is, what it means, and what we do with it. When we consider the eclectic assortment of fitness activities and pursuits, when we mine individual experiences and collective actions, when we merge the critical and the creative, when we employ the personal and political, American fitness demonstrates its transformative power and potential. Fitness is, after all, complex and layered and experienced differently for each of us even as we are all confined by dominant culture's expectations and mechanisms.

This book—this critical and creative exploration—brings together a variety of aspects of fitness and cultural critique. My interdisciplinary academic methods are akin to the fitness concept of cross-training. I combine creative, academic, and practical approaches to understanding fitness. I bring together a mosaic: short essays, academic inquiries, poetry, creative non-fiction, memoir, choreography, personal experience, observation, character sketches, social and cultural critique. Literal and figurative, reflective and prospective, this book asks us to question our preconceived notions about ourselves and about our ideas of fitness; it aims to inspire us to continue to develop meanings and modes for feminist fitness, for empowerment, and for critique. It asks us to think about fitness as a metaphor, as an individual pursuit, as an exploitative practice, as a community endeavor, and as an industry. It asks us to think about the ways in which fitness is an important part of our lives that cannot and should not be sacrificed or denied. It asks us to think about how we each define fitness in theory and as we embody our ideas. It asks us to think about what "fitness" is to us and to think about how we can bring "fitness" to others.[1]

* * *

I have been a fitness instructor for nearly fifteen years, teaching, and attending a variety of fitness classes and fitness trainings and workshops. I have also been an academic during this time, pursuing an M.A. in English and a Ph.D. in American Studies and holding several academic teaching positions in these fields. So, in addition to teaching step, kickboxing, muscle conditioning, Pilates, yoga, belly dancing, and cardio dance, I also teach classes in English, women's studies, and American studies. Sometimes these worlds coalesce. And recently, after years of being encouraged to keep these spheres separate, I have worked to bring them together by bringing academia into fitness and fitness into academia. As the editors of *Women and Exercise: The Body, Health and Consumerism* point out, the assumptions about exercise as being non-feminist means that "many feminists 'hide' or 'segregate' their possible exercise lives from their critical work" (6); the same is more generally true in many fields, including those I was trained in: American studies, comparative ethnic studies, sociology, English, and women's studies. And this purposeful omittance, this denial of work that shaped me personally and professionally, felt wrong. On paper, and as a professional, I felt incomplete. Fitness stayed at the edges even though it was a key part of my self.

After being trained as a fitness instructor in an academic setting the last semester of my undergraduate education, I taught fitness classes throughout graduate school and in addition to each academic teaching position I have had after graduate school. And now that I have a tenure-track job, with colleagues who support my work in fitness and do not see it as counter to academia, I have been able to grow this work in many directions. I have begun to teach fitness in academic workshops. I have included belly dancing — theory and practice and critique — into my "Introduction to Women's Studies" classes and in a 300-level American studies and women's studies class: "Culture, Consciousness, and Community." I have presented my work on feminist fitness at a local women's studies conference and as creative/critical workshop at the National Women's Studies Association conference. I have developed community workshops and have offered special classes as fundraisers for scholarships. I have invited my students to my classes at the local YMCA, and I have connected with colleagues across campuses. These are some of the experiences I consider here.

These professional developments have also been encouraged by a book that I came across when I began to develop my vision of fitness in academia. When I found *My Life at the Gym*, edited by Jo Malin, I felt like I had found myself again. Here, in print, was a book that supported my merging of feminism and fitness, of academia and fitness. For Jo Malin, this was the first merging of her academic life and her fitness life. I could identify. Here were stories and critiques and musings and questionings from all sorts of women who also love (or love/hate or tolerate) fitness and find ways to fit fitness into their professional (and largely academic) lives. And here were women who felt passionately about the positive impacts of fitness in their lives. This book unleashed the last remnants of self-doubt and fear that hovered between the merging spaces of my life in fitness and my life in academia. It inspired me to create an American studies/women's studies class: "American Fitness: Culture, Community, and Transformation." It also led me to find Tara Brabazon's "Fitness is a Feminist Issue" and, later, Eileen Kennedy and Pirkko Markula's *Women and Exercise. My Life at the Gym* helped me give myself permission to write this book and "Fitness Is a Feminist Issue" provided a strong academic foundation. I blend these academic explorations with popular sources, and my own practical knowledge and critical readings of culture, in an attempt to create a book that can straddle the popular and the academic and interrupt and rearrange the binaries that rule both of these spheres.[2]

* * *

Women and Fitness in American Culture takes fitness as a malleable shifting reality, as a concept to be explored through a particular set of tools and experiences that are inherently feminist, evolving and reflective. It questions the ways in which mainstream ideas of health and fitness have shaped our personal lives and our social lives, our institutions and our culture. Each of the five chapters builds upon and connects to the others, and an organic structure emerges. Disciplines cross, the past informs the present, and the popular complements the academic. Between and among chapters there are related themes and different versions of the same fitness concepts or experiences. The chapters build from definition to application to reflection to transformation. There is no chronological historical exploration, only a few pointed discussions of past research precedents or past trends. Instead, myriad fitness threads are woven together. Each part, or each piece, stands alone; but together, all of the parts create a whole — a moving body, a moving mind/body.

Chapter One, "Tensions: Form and Function," explores a variety of literal and figurative tensions beginning with the idea of "fitness" itself and the gendered expectations that we have in terms of fitness. This chapter examines the terrain of fitness in America, from the personal experiences of my childhood to the ways fitness functions in industry and through popular culture. Some of the assumed connections to fitness are more closely examined — the affiliations of health, sport, and science, the kinds of spaces fitness needs, and the inescapable topic of body image. I also consider the language of fitness — the ways in which we shape translations of movement into language and the ways in which the language of fitness is mathematically structured. I briefly sketch out some of the "transformative innovators" whose ideas about fitness have transformed the industry as well as individuals; following this introduction to transformative innovators, each chapter includes sketches of fitness movers: innovators, instructors, and participants. The form and function of fitness are always in tension — a form that takes on patriarchy's demands while it simultaneously functions to empower and ignite.

Chapter Two, "Tools and Trade" balances academic and kinesthetic approaches to fitness as it delves deeper into aspects of work and the nature of fitness as work — the exploitation and the empowerment. These are a trade off. I consider fitness as a trade and as a set of skills. I include the skilled workers of fitness through sketches of fitness instructors. I build a toolbox that blurs boundaries and methodologies between fitness and academia. I also consider fitness through my professional trade — through my work as an academic, as a professor. Anticipating Chapter Three, I provide an overview of some of the academic perspectives on fitness as well the feminist foundations of fitness in academia, foundations that are fundamental to this book as well as to developing fitness outside the demands of mainstream definitions. I consider the political nature of fitness as well as the unexpected connections that we might find between fitness and academia. For instance, I consider the controversial icon Jane Fonda, and the coincidental origins of the "aerobics" revolution during the revolutionary justice movements of the late 1960s. The work of fitness includes the work that we must do to maintain a commitment to fitness and the compromises we must make in order to achieve, let alone maintain, fitness. I also question whether fitness might better enable us to serve others in educational and activist contexts. Finally, I consider fitness and consciousness through a key metaphor for fitness instructors — the wearing of many hats — and a complementary concept understood in academic terms through theories of critical consciousness.

There are many incarnations of feminist fitness and these shift from location to location, space to space. Chapter Three, "Toward a Theory of Feminist

Fitness," begins to explicitly discuss and critique the idea and practice of feminist fitness. I explore some of the ways in which fitness is a subject of women's studies and how fitness manifests itself in feminist ways. In introductory classes in women's studies, I introduce students to belly dancing as a form of fitness but also as a kind of consciousness, and as a way of connecting the West with the East; I share some of the critical approaches and student interpretations from this work. I also include some consideration of the many ways of connecting people through fitness, whether this is through the more traditionally "feminine" outlets of dance or the solitary and communal pursuits of running, biking, or walking. In the last section I consider the creative/critical approach to fitness that I explore throughout the book and begin to theorize in more detail in this chapter.

Chapter Four, "Edges/Bodies and Minds" explores the edges of my fitness world/culture — the parts that are sharp, unhealed. Love makes fitness more whole and more complicated, and I struggle to lift the weight of generations of women in my family and friends who have been unhappy with their bodies. The perceptions of "fat" and the marginalization of older and larger women, from life as well as the gym, are considered more deeply than their outside edges. I explore the ways in which fitness provides access to spirituality in a variety of forms. I return to many early topics, approaching from the edge rather than the center. I reconsider body image and disordered eating through mother/father issues and through the idea of consumption. Through sketches I highlight the people who populate fitness classes, in all their glorious variety, rather than focus on the instructor or class style or brand. Fitness also pulls us back from the edges and heals rifts. It transforms our bodies, our minds, and our lives. Thus, I explore fitness as a healing art, as a pathway to a more conscious, more centered, more balanced, more whole person. And the edges that separate body and mind are, I hope, welded more closely together.

Chapter Five, "Transformations" reminds us of the power and potential power of feminist reconsiderations of fitness. Here I return to some of the subjects covered in previous chapters and transform the conversation as I consider the possibility of developing critical, even oppositional, consciousness through fitness. With this critical consciousness, Chapter Five offers feminist analyses and examples of transformation. I also consider the power that fitness has had in transforming my life and my work, particularly discovering the power of dance. This transformation further transforms my teaching as I literally and figuratively change directions — teaching facing the class, rather than facing away, facing a mirror. The transformative aspects of these modes of fitness offers mind/body transformations for individuals and communities, but also the possibility of critical transformations of culture and society, of the fitness industry, and the relationship of fitness to the more "serious" pursuits of life. Ultimately, without fitness we have no life. With fitness we always have, at the very least, the potential for mind/body empowerment, and, at the very least, gaining or shifting perspective. We also have a source of pleasure that can ignite our passion.

* * *

John F. Kennedy gave fitness a cultural and historical relevance and value (a legacy, perhaps). Kenneth Cooper rationalized and systematized fitness. Jane Fonda made it fun and Wii Fit made it convenient, simple, and interactive. American fitness has transformed over time and has transformed us. Further transformation — an embrace of mind/body fitness — begins with critical and creative explorations of this thing, this state, this idea we call "fitness." *Women and Exercise* concludes with the thought that the collective findings of its chapters "foreshadow women's attempts to step away from the limitations of ... fitness to define their own engagement in exercise and physical activity" (21). This is where *Women and Fitness in American Culture* begins. I step away from these limitations — provide practical and imaginative explorations of fitness — and I hope that women (and men) will not only "[re]define their own engagement," but also find ways to contribute to a radical rethinking of what fitness means to us individually and collectively.

The Warm Up

My eyes open. The music is in my head. It wakes my body. Excitement and anticipation. I crave the stomp, slide and pull up. I crave the hip circles, snake arms, shakes, and shimmies. I feel my body loosen and center. Once I get through my work — long hours focused, magnanimous, multi-tasking — my reward is movement. Transformation.

I am tired. It's been a long day, a long week, a long semester. I have to put on my instructor hat and inspire a room full of women. I crave a nap and a pizza. I don't feel like teaching tonight. The music starts and my mood is transformed. My body moves with new energy. I feel alive and lucky to be able to move with a group of people who have also set aside their long day, long week, stressful lives — people who enjoy movement. I remember all the reasons why I am there. I remind myself. I am transformed.

I am stiff and my body aches. All of the variations of what we could do in class that day quickly run through my head. Will the room be cold today? Will we have enough blocks? The women roll in and roll out their mats. The yoga poses flow from memory and take shape in new combinations. We challenge our minds and our bodies. We ignore outside distractions like the chanting of the drill sergeant in the gym on the other side of the thin door or the making of our to-do lists. We balance and stretch and build strength. Three days a week begin with yoga and they are the best days. For the rest of the day a feeling of strength, well-being, and relaxation follows me. I have been transformed.

I am slightly dizzy, almost intoxicated. The music ends but I do not want to move. I want to do it all again. A routine — complete and perfect. The pieces all fall into place. My body is completely relaxed. My mind has stopped harping on this or that. I have managed not to think for an hour. I have been set free.

My colleague snickers as I relate my summer activities — not much: taught summer school, taught yoga. He laughs because he thinks, and says, "white people can't do yoga" and because he sees me as nothing but another liberal white girl who adopts the spiritual practices of "the other" uncritically and without an appreciation for the origins and "true" forms.[3] He does not know me. And he doesn't know yoga. He does not know the power of yoga in this world. But my practice has only begun a process that is in perpetual motion. He does not see my critiques or transformations, my ability to empower. I push against the edges.

I nervously clear the chairs from the conference room, the typical hotel chairs and carpet, crumbs and empty coffee cups, crushed M&Ms. I wonder if anyone will show up. A small group slowly gathers, expectant and maybe a bit nervous. *As nervous as I am?* I have to clear more space than I expected. (My mother helps me, observes, supports.) This workshop is nothing like the many panels and workshops that fill the National Women's Studies Association's conference program. It is something different. This workshop is the first I have done outside my local studios. I rush through my introduction. We begin the activity — a feminist fitness class — and my legs feel a bit weak, my feet ungrounded on the new surface of hotel carpet. I find my groove as we move together. We laugh and play. And they enjoy it. They are engaged. I am drained and energized.

My memory consistently fails me. Fuzzy memories and an imperfect photographic memory, I recall pages and places, ideas and patterns, but few details. I remember spaces and movement. I remember faces more often than names. My mind prefers abstraction, connection, reference — the big picture. My body, on the other hand, locks memory in movement. Routines, sequences, songs, choreography — in part and in whole — clutter my brain but are neatly, calmly, perfectly expressed through my body. I move and the words come to me without effort. The music begins and the movements and verbal cues and physical cues flow effortlessly. Over a decade of work/ing (out), of building routines, fishing for moves, balancing variables — all are embedded in bones and flesh and consciousness. It is a critical and creative transformation from music to movement, from mind to body, from movement to language. From individual to group.

I am transformed.

And I have set myself free.

ONE

Tensions: Form and Function

Fitness Forms: Toward a Definition

> *Fitness, according to the American Medical Association (AMA)*: Physical fitness is "the general capacity to adapt favorably to physical effort; an individual is physically fit when he is able to meet both the usual and unusual demands on daily life, safely and effectively."
>
> *Generally, five components can determine overall physical fitness:* Muscular Strength, Flexibility, Cardiovascular Health, Muscular Endurance, Lean/Fat Body Mass. Some exercise scientists add: balance, coordination, agility, speed, and power to this list.
>
> *Fitness, according to the American Council on Exercise (ACE):* A person who is physically fit: "has an enhanced functional capacity that allows for a high quality of life." A high quality of life is described as: "overall positive feeling and enthusiasm for life" and "the ability to do enriching and enjoyable activities without fatigue."[1]
>
> "There is no standard level of fitness.... The key is that the body must be able to meet daily physical challenges, with the capacity to stretch and extend when circumstances demand it."
>
> — Tara Brabazon, "Fitness Is a Feminist Issue" (72)

In 1956 President Eisenhower established the President's Council on Youth Fitness and this council was renamed by President Kennedy in 1963 as the President's Council on Physical Fitness, to address adults' fitness as well. In 1968 this council was shifted to Physical Fitness and Sports. (Kolata 43) In 2010 the council was renamed by President Obama as the President's Council on Fitness, Sports, and Nutrition. This shift certainly speaks to the shifts that have taken place in American culture after World War II.[2] Dr. Kenneth Cooper's work in the 1960s sought to "determine the relationship of physical fitness and health" (viii) and aimed to give people some idea of how much activity to do, what kind of activity to do, and how long to do such activity. In the preface to *Aerobics*, Senator William Proxmire reminds readers that

13

Cooper's formula is "simple" and "easy" and argues that this book "will do more for the health and longevity of Americans than any other medical discovery or achievement of the year" (viii). Cooper's *Aerobics* was also excerpted in *This Week Magazine* and *Reader's Digest* and a Book-of-the-Month Club edition was published in the summer of 1968. Clearly his ideas of fitness were marketed to the masses. Americans like "simple" and "easy" even as we might recognize, as Lt. General Bohannon does in his introduction to *Aerobics*, that "the word 'fitness,' as applied to physical conditioning, has been an ill-defined, confusing term." We might recognize "reasonable muscular development" and "functional flexibility," perhaps even "psychological well-being" (ix). But fitness is simplified in popular consciousness and we miss the nuances.

Despite the fact that scientists, athletes, and fitness professionals have expanded on these early definitions and studies, and organizations like the AMA and ACE have given us the kind of concise definition that Bohannon encouraged, our concerns when it comes to physical fitness have not changed drastically. Senator Proxmire notes in his preface that "death from heart disease is the number one killer in American today" and that there is a general inability to pass fitness tests, a lack of time devoted to "physical exertion" and a connection between disability and "excessive inactivity. All of these are conditions that are true today. As Tara Brabazon points out in her 2006 article, "The health benefits of raising the heart rate, sweating and increasing cardiovascular fitness are ignored by the bulk of the American population" (71). Does this mean that we have lost the battle? Maybe. But perhaps we have set ourselves up for failure in the ways we have imagined, and engaged, in this "battle." Perhaps it's not a battle at all.

Fitness is a term that encompasses a variety of meanings. It is both more simple and more complicated than we tend to think it is. Many fitness-related books that I cite here begin by defining the term, simplifying it, codifying it. Sometimes recognizing its complexity. Scientific studies have explored fitness and health, athletic ability, and other measurable yet contestable facts of fitness. At the same times, fitness programs have emerged to discipline our minds and bodies. Fitness products have followed to aid us in our quest for fit perfection. And fitness representations have linked all sorts of things — particularly beauty and appearance and desirability — to fitness. Cooper sought a simple, straight-forward formula for fitness (exemplified through his chapter titles: the problem, the key, the exercises, the test, the system, the rules and the goal) that could be followed by anyone desiring better physical conditioning. His program's goals were relatively simple and were presented through accessible, entertaining, authoritative writing and a logical plan. "If you follow the point system and get enough of the right kind of exercise, it will produce many wonderful changes in your body that are cumulatively known as the 'training effect'" or "the whole goal of endurance exercise" (12). Similar models have been replicated, expanded, and enhanced by many different programs and, yet, as a nation, "fitness" continues to elude us. Thus, it may just be time to reconsider the terms of our pursuit.

The best definition of fitness comes from a collage of understanding. Brabazon's definition of fitness builds from the "standard" and "physical" to consider one's "capacity to *stretch and extend* when circumstances demand it" (my emphasis). We are fit when we can adapt, flow, and grow. On a larger scale, fitness is molded through an exploration of the shades of meaning in society and culture and through global comparisons and implications. It is also discovered through a personal understanding of one's own body in context — its potential and real limitations. Fitness is understood by its theoretical underpinnings and by its practice in a variety of settings. Because fitness is also a personal state of being, it is found in a variety of forms that might not mesh with industry standards or working definitions. But because this is not the vision of health and wellness that we are sold through a variety of cultural texts, it is not the way we are used to thinking about "fitness." These are some of the shades of fitness that this book explores.

* * *

Fitness is a loaded word that holds a weight of assumptions about the body. It is a term that has been used, historically, to create dangerous programs like the "Fitter Family" programs of the Eugenics movement or "revolutionary" approaches to fitness that will be further explored in this book. Expectations of body size have been disguised as discussions about "fitness" and height/weight ratio charts dictate one set of rigid ratios, discounting a number of factors. And, as Brabazon notes, height/weight charts were designed by the life insurance industry "to evaluate the risk of prospective clients" (73).[3] The irony of the term "fitness," as applied to the emaciated bodies of models or the hyper-pumped bodies of athletes and body builders is "American fitness."

Gina Kolata both reinforces and challenges what "fitness" is through her investigative journalistic style in her 2003 book, *Ultimate Fitness: The Quest for Truth About Exercise and Health*. As a science writer, Kolata examines the research; as a reporter, she focuses on people's stories — including her own. Each chapter hovers around a central question, theme, or representation of fitness and ends with a series of questions as one exploration leads to the next. Kolata seems particularly focused on appearance and performance. Even so, the picture she paints reveals the interconnected layers of American fitness and the vast amount of information that we must sift through if we want to understand this subject. She gives a history and an exploration of science that is shaped by her passion — weights and Spinning. Somewhat surprisingly, she concludes that while people exercise to improve health, appearance, and performance, pleasure is, ultimately, why people exercise or at least why they keep exercising. (266–7) Part of my argument here is that the "pleasure" of exercise is an untapped resource for an understanding of, and practice of, "American Fitness." Pleasure is key, but pleasure, in American culture, is variegated, mediated, skewed and sublimated.

* * *

At times I use "fitness" to generalize and at other times I use it to refer specifically to a common understanding of "aerobics" or "exercise." Sometimes I use the term to challenge what it means; I shift the context or question assumptions. Other times I assume that my reader knows that "fitness" stands for more than what the word means narrowly. But my fitness bias is clear throughout this book. My experience comes from a subset of the larger whole of fitness — "group fitness." The term group fitness, Brabazon explains, is the term used more recently to refer to what has been previously known as "aerobics." The term "group fitness" is usually reserved for a specific kind of fitness class. A group fitness class can be of any variety of type of fitness class, taught by one instructor (or sometimes more) to a small (or sometimes large) group of people. Step or Step Aerobics is group fitness. Yoga is group fitness. Bootcamp is group fitness. Group fitness is manufactured through companies like Body Training Systems, Zumba, and Les Mills as well as YogaFit, Power Yoga, Nia, and many others. It is created organically by trained professionals or passionate amateurs. It is experienced individually and collectively. It keeps us in a mainstream American mold but also empowers us to break free of this mold.

And group fitness has evolved over the decades. Kolata explores a longer history — from ancient Greece through the present, noting that post–World War II fitness expanded as "in the late seventies, the health-club movement, which grew out of the aerobics movement, saw a marketing opportunity" (226). Brabazon sums up the last few decades of American group fitness:

> The 1970s was a decade of tough fitness — no pain, no gain. The 1980s was a time of designer exercise, a balancing of cream cocktails with step aerobics. The 1990s appropriated orientalist discourses to affirm wellness, whole body fitness and yoga. Through the 2000s, exercise has been consumed almost as readily as pre-packaged food through the Les Mills group fitness programmes [sic] [66].

Here this historical trajectory seems simple and straight forward. We can see these shifts and critique the ways in which the changes in the fitness industry have also mirrored the changes in our culture and political economy. As Kolata notes, in 2002 there were more than 17,000 health clubs in the U.S. and 32.8 million health club members. These are, Kolata notes, "a fragment of the exercise business that has grown up in my adult lifetime" (253). We can see the ways in which women have been at the center and margins of these shifts simultaneously. But fitness is certainly more complicated than all of this. Brabazon further explains that aerobics has multiple origins and cannot be contained within one category (67). This hybrid nature of aerobics, or "fitness" more generally, is important to a larger understanding of the importance of fitness as a physical reality and a metaphorical way of understanding American fitness.

Slightly abstracted, "group fitness" is also community fitness, it is a form of fitness that can be offered almost anywhere and at almost any time. It can be a kind of fitness that is free or one that is provided for a fee. It can be proscriptive or transformative, and sometimes both at the same time. Fitness is also a term that holds the potential for a redefinition of itself—it is a concept constantly in process. Fitness is molded by trends and traditions, fads and fantasies. But "fitness" is also contested by groups and individuals who challenge dominant ideas of fitness and find a form of fitness that nourishes mind/body and even community. As metaphor, certainly fitness holds much meaning for how we live our lives and see our bodies. Strength, flexibility, balance, endurance, and agility all offer important means for survival and prosperity.

Fitness, like many other pursuits that require time, money, and resources of all kinds, is often a privilege or a luxury or is at least associated with access to time and money. But fitness can be more simple and more complex and the idea of fitness is bigger than this view allows it to be. The privileges of fitness are a reality that closely mirror those other kinds of privileges and inequalities in American culture. As Louise Mansfield argues, "the tendency, then, in contemporary Western life, is for people to perceive that their bodies should be worked-on, and worked-out as a means of representing and expressing the individual self" (81). We can find power (and perhaps empowerment) through the manipulation of our bodies, but too often we are taught that our outward appearance has the most value. Tara Brabazon explains further, "Certainly, women are transforming the self into a project. It is a negotiated self, a site of both anxiety and display" (67). And a whole industry—a set of American institutions—encourage us in this anxiety-laden work. Sports represent uber-fitness while media represents thinness in anorexic proportions. Men seek to take up space; women disappear.[4]

Fitness is also often associated with and understood through a lens of masculinity. Some women are afraid of "bulking up" or looking "like men" if they use weights.[5] Or maybe strength is not even on our radar. Even as these women may be desirous of "results," the results they are most often concerned with (following culture) are weight loss, not muscles (*Women and Exercise* 128). Trainers often take up a "boot camp" approach and weakness is associated with women as a motivating factor, for instance, throwing "like a girl" or, worse, being weak like a "pussy."[6] Our fitness standards are often based upon assumptions about men's strength and women's grace and flexibility. But while there is some biological basis for different fitness-related activities, these gendered assumptions are stereotypes that have been reinforced through culture and media. Despite differences of sex — averages of size, strength, height, build, shape — fitness goals need not be gender-specific. Strength, balance, flexibility, and cardiovascular endurance are universal signs of fit bodies; it is our culture that is gendered.

* * *

One need not look far for an example of gendered expectations regarding fitness; they saturate our culture. Most fitness magazines or online sources rely on gendered stereotypes. For instance, an August 2012 headline on MSN Fitbie announced the "Fitness Bucket List" — the fitness goals that everyone should try to achieve in their lifetime — and had two links, one to a bucket list for men and one for women. These two separate, but related, articles were written by fitness reporter Myatt Murphy, who is credited with having his work appear in "innumerable magazines and on-line"; however, it is clear that his work is about men's fitness, and these two articles reflect this bias while they also provide a glimpse at the way in which gender shapes our fitness culture.

In the introduction Murphy illustrates the ways in which masculinity can be confining and demanding for men: "There are a few fitness goals that every guy knows he needs to achieve within his lifetime." The women's list assumes superficiality in our relationship to fitness (we want to look good in a certain dress or a new bathing suit); the men's list assumes that men have specialized knowledge of the fitness expectations that they "need to achieve." And accomplishing the bucket list goals is set up as a challenge; these are exercises that come with bragging rights. Women should "strive for" our bucket list goals "at least once — just so your body can thank you for it later!" Just how our body will "thank us for it later" is not clear from this statement, but the assumption might be that these fitness goals are more than just an achievement to strive for, but also a means toward feeling better in our bodies. Murphy even implies that we might not even be able to do these things on the list, but as long as we try, even if it's only once, it's okay to fail. These are quite different messages about men's and women's fitness goals and the idea of the bucket list. Interestingly, the author recognizes that some of the men's goals are just as frivolous as the women's goals of that perfect dress; both sexes can, after all, flaunt their bodies in different, and totally gendered, ways. But it's more complicated.

Not surprisingly, two of the goals for men target upper-body strength. The others target body fat (waist circumference), speed, and flexibility. The fact that he includes flexibility is a promising sign; however, the only "goal" here is to be able to touch your toes and the reason behind this goal is that "having that kind of flexibility that can prevent unnecessary back pain caused from tight, stiff lower back muscles and hamstrings." This is relevant to men and an important goal to include; however, when we compare this to the last goal for women, "hold tree pose for 60 seconds," the differences are illuminating. On the women's bucket list, holding tree pose is representative of having a yoga practice as a part of one's fitness routine. Murphy writes: "the end result: you build functional strength that trains your muscles to work collectively, which can improve your performance in any everyday activity or sport." This is an important fitness goal for men and women and, yet, for men the importance of flexibility is shrunken down to the elimination or management of back pain while for women the importance of balance is conflated with "functional strength."

Murphy's "Fitness Bucket List" provides an instructive example for beginning to think about the gendered expectations of American fitness and how these gendered expectations, like other kinds of gendered expectations, help to shape how we think men and women *should* be.[7] Men should be strong and competitive; women should be sculpted and social. Men should do; women should try. Murphy replicates these expectations but provides women with a more meaningful list of goals. Fitness expectations for men are well-entrenched and have set our national agenda and shaped our collective fitness consciousness. These expectations deserve to be unpacked and rearranged. And re-created. Perhaps when we consider how women change the fitness equation we might not need a "bucket list." We can all work toward "functional strength."

"Fitness," then, is most often abstract, but it is also a fundamentally embodied idea and ideal. This "ideal" concept is problematic in the ways in which we are taught to think about perfection and the body's most trained and maintained physical capabilities. Instead, this fitness concept as ideal is specific to each body — to abilities, to time and place, to genetics, to preference, to the possibilities. And it is an ideal that engages body and mind as well as collective power and critical consciousness ... if we want it to.

* * *

Exploring the themes, terms, and figures that dominate American fitness, this first part of *Women and Fitness in American Culture* attempts to layer a groundwork for a more nuanced understanding of fitness. We need to better understand what "American fitness" is before we can transform it. I consider pop culture — the realm of the most accepted definitions of fitness — as well as the fads and gadgets that help shape this fitness terrain. In addition, I consider the limitations of manufactured fitness, the pre-programmed routines that make promises of better bodies. I consider the fitness affiliations of health, sport, and science and how these all help to shape the way in which we understand fitness. Through poetry I lay a foundation for understanding movement, and in memoir I share some of my preparation from girlhood. I consider the language of fitness the idea of movement. In exploration related to later complications, I also consider body image and eating disorders as they plague the world of fitness. Finally, a look at fitness spaces provides a literal and figurative view of where we pursue fitness.

The various forms that fitness takes also have a variety of functions, whether these are mechanical, kinesthetic functions or more ethereal functions. The tensions emerge when form does not follow function or function does not follow form. When fitness practices become dangerous, when the structured confines of mainstream expectations are challenged, when movement is redefined, tensions grind.

Lessons from Girlhood: Developing Skills and Passion

I often tell people that I never would have imagined that I would grow up to be a fitness instructor. Me: fat, shy, bookworm. What I imagined for myself was limited by the role models I saw and the skills I knew I did or didn't have. But this is only part of the truth (and it is a biased truth). The truth is I never imagined I would be a fitness instructor just like I never imagined that I would be a college professor. The former was just not me and the latter I didn't even know existed as a possible profession. And even though I saw myself as fat, felt myself as shy, and knew I enjoyed books more than most other activities, these attributes were shaped by the limitations of circumstance and vision.

But fitness was always a part of my life, most obviously through sports. Mine was the first generation of girls to be encouraged in sports en masse. My father's love of sports and my mother's knowledge that sports were especially important for a number of developmental skills — not just physical but mental and social too — was the impetus for my participation in organized sports leagues, playing soccer and softball for my entire childhood and soccer and volleyball through my first three years of high school. Sports were a struggle and I found my niche in different ways — sometimes aiming to inspire other players, sometimes aiming to be the reliable defender, always finding a sense of empowerment through the workings of team efforts to survive, let alone win. My father hoped for college scholarships and my mother hoped for well-rounded children.

Sports have certainly influenced my abilities as a fitness instructor. Other activities for the well-rounded, middle-class child — dance, gymnastics, and piano lessons — have also coalesced in my fitness-teaching skills. I was never really very talented at any of these. A mediocre dancer without the patience for precision or for memorizing other people's choreography but with a sense of the beat and what I later learned was called "musicality." A gymnast without natural flexibility and without the kind of fearlessness that allows one to learn a back walkover, for instance. A piano player with an ear to pick out tunes and to memorize songs but without the patience to read sheet music or to learn the coordination between the independent left and right hands. And on the sports field, well, I worked my ass off but we never won much more than a few games a season. I was consistent and smart but not spectacular, and the sporting world likes superstars. I was a fierce competitor, finding some sense of a desire to prove myself and for my team to prove itself. But I was never surprised, or devastated, or even much affected by the many defeats my teams suffered. I was also never much impressed by the occasional winning seasons that I felt I contributed very little to. Someone had to lose and all the other stuff — the pain, sweat, tears, struggles, camaraderie — all seemed worth it, regardless.

While all of these mandatory childhood activities contributed to my skill set as an instructor — my stamina, my ability to recognize and count musical phrases, my love of choreography, my creativity and flexibility, my storehouse of movements — there were other experiences that led me, consciously or not, to pursue the unreachable dream of "fitness instructor."

Some of these are fond childhood memories.... My mother in leotard, tights, and legwarmers and her random, repeated chant from Jane Fonda:

"and repeat to the left and to the right." The Mickey's "Mousekercise" records that I would exercise to as a child, reaching into the sky with Porky Pig for the invisible treats above our heads and trying to get Uncle Scrooge's money. I can still see the scenes vividly in my head today and remember many of the tunes and lyrics. And my desire to be beautiful. I saw women in dance and fitness as beautiful and while I never ever imagined that I really *looked* like them, I often imagined that I was them and I often *felt* beautiful while in movement, even if that feeling was only fleeting or barely conscious. This feeling was very different from other physical activities; organized sports and physical education classes in grades six through nine emphasized running, calisthenics, and skills. Growing up in southern California, we did not have a gym until high school and, thus, all of our physical education activities took place outside and with very limited equipment. (For instance, we trained for a track meet mocking the movement of the high jump because we did not have anything to jump over or land on.) Part of the reason I returned to dance classes in junior high was the association of dance with beauty and desirability. I was comfortable with sports and shy with dance. I wanted to be comfortable with dance. My friend Annie and I took a Jazz and Modern dance class from a eccentric dance teacher that we knew from church. We would wear the most ridiculous outfits including torn t-shirts and bikini bottoms over panty hose rolled down to reveal our bellies. Our dance classes were short-lived for a variety of reasons. For a time I really wanted to be a dancer in music videos, but my total lack of talent or flexibility and my perceived lack of beauty quickly made this dream fade.

These are the experiences that lead to the inspiration, the passion for fitness. All of those skills, all of those activities that made me "well-rounded" also provided the foundations for excellence in this under-recognized art form. But all of these skills — near perfect cueing, an ear for music, a talent for putting movement to music — would be nothing without the passion for fitness that grows from a variety of sources like dance and sports and is expressed through a variety of fitness modes.

During the latter part of my childhood, as I struggled toward adulthood, I was introduced to the more formal world of group fitness. This was quite different from the "fitness" I had been introduced to through sports and P.E. classes. One of my physical education teachers in 9th grade held an aerobics class for us during P.E. class and it was so much better than running! When I decided not to play sports my senior year (a difficult decision that greatly disappointed my father), I started taking Jazzercise and step classes with my mother. I enjoyed being in these spaces filled with women, focused and joyful. I loved the way I felt during/after class. I enjoyed watching the dynamics of fitness classes — who claimed what space, who filled the empty time before class stretching or sitting or gossiping. I found the choreography easy to pick up and pleasurable to follow. There was a different kind of competition than what I found on the soccer field; some people competed with other class members and others competed with the instructor. Some of us were not competing at all. And I could compete with myself— remembering the steps, committing to the patterns, pushing myself beyond where I thought I could go.

I always admired the instructors and saw them as perfect, dynamic, magnetic. Untouchable. At a women's gym, waiting for class to begin, I tried not to stare too intently as the regular instructor coached her trainee before class. I could not tear my attention away. I had not thought about group fitness as something that you learned in that way. I had imagined intense trainings, tests, serious memorization and repetitive practice. Or, I imagined they just knew how to do it innately. But, I had not really thought much about it at all. And I certainly did not think of it as something I could do. At seventeen I had a path planned out — college, graduate school, career, marriage and children. I planned to have it all. I certainly did not imagine that I would be a fitness instructor.

But throughout my childhood I had imagined all sorts of impossible or improbable careers. I actually thought at one time that I might be a singer or a dancer, a pastor, a lawyer, a doctor, a writer. I was intent on finding out who I would *be* when I grew up and that identity was completely wrapped up in *what* I would be. I certainly would not be a college athlete or any kind of religiously-affiliated leader. My mom would make suggestions based upon what I was good at (always something where I would use my brain first and foremost). And while it was mentioned that I would be a good teacher (of some kind; I assumed, of high school), no one would have suggested that I become a fitness instructor. Since I prefer to follow my own suggestions and inclinations, this is probably a good thing. It just kind of happened because I enjoyed fitness classes and thought I could make some money while I went to school. But is has also happened with a lot of hard work, dedication, practice, humility, confidence, and love.

Fitness is a safe space for me, a safe space to express myself through my body, to merge the disconnect. In fitness I am strong and successful, but I can also be playful and sexy. I can lead and I can follow. I can be the professor as much as I am the girl with the rolled down pantyhose. In fitness, I am confident in my skills and comfortable in my body. These are lessons that weren't quite learned in girlhood, but in girlhood is where they originated. And it has taken time for these lessons to develop into conscious knowledge and practical applications. The process continues, forms and reforms.

Movement

> Movement means transformation —
> Social, cultural, physical —
> A promise of a better future
> A different way to be
>
> Movement inspires transformation —
> Of bodies, ideas, policies
> Political and corporal
> Shifting sand or muscle
>
> Old wounds may be healed
> New wounds may open
> And boundaries stretch
> Beyond body or mind
>
> We may stumble in our movements
> Clashing measures
> Failing to measure up
> We may repeat the same mistakes
>
> We commit movement to memory
> Repeat it
> Enough to memorize it
> Repeat it enough to forget it was
>
> Memory
> And remember
> it is perpetual —
> Movement.

Pop Culture: Icons, Products and Representations

"PUMA has been in the Helps-You-Look-Good™ business since 1948. /We know what we're doing. People in magazines wear this stuff. Fashion people, sporty people. People who don't have to wear a suit everyday./So, we know it works."
　　　　— Blurb on a tag that came on a pair of PUMA shoes

While my PUMA shoes are darn cute, I am far more concerned about whether they will provide me with proper support during class. My main goal is not to look good but to end class without my feet, and the rest of my body by extension, hurting. I actually prefer Saucony over all other athletic shoes, but they grip the floor too well for Group Groove. I have to have a shoe with a smoother tread for fitness dancing. So a smooth surface, comfort, and then style are what I consider. (Finding comfort, affordability, and functionality in a sweatshop-free product seem nearly impossible.) Even though

I never wear a suit, I am hardly one of those "fashion people" or even "sporty people" that PUMA is referring to. But I sometimes buy their shoes. And sometimes people tell me how cute they are. This is a surface of fitness — the products of pop culture that dominate our imaginations and shape our experiences with fitness. As Kolata notes, Cooper "set the stage for health clubs, aerobics classes, personal trainers, bodysculpting, special exercise gear, and magazines and books promising health and beauty through fitness" (46). There's nothing wrong with looking good; we often feel good as well. But the business of looking good is a bit more complicated when we look at the bigger picture.

Bodies — mostly thin, mostly white, scantily-clad bodies — dominate the image of "fitness" in popular culture. We have the belief that thin, young, tan bodies are "better bodies."[8] We think they can do more and, really, who cares what they can *do* as long as they are more enjoyable to look at? We also make the assumption that, for men, muscles equal no brains and, for women, muscles equal a threat, a desire to be masculine, if not a man. As Kennedy and Markula argue, "in popular media texts, looking good (the ideal body) and feeling good (health) become closely intertwined" (3). In addition to this superficial view of the healthy body, The American Psychological Association (APA) has stated that studies show that *all media forms* sexualize women and girls — music, magazine, internet, video games, movies, and television all have in common the sexualization and objectification of women and girls. In "Keep Your Clothes On! Fit and Sexy Through Striptease Aerobics" Magdalena Petersson McIntyre describes that sexualized forms of aerobics need to be "seen in the light of a normalization of striptease and pornography that has taken place since the 1990s ... porn has turned chic and pole dancing has been repackaged as fitness" (250). Because this "normalization" is expressed through girls' and women's bodies, the connections in popular culture between sexual desirability and physical fitness are intertwined.

While popular culture remains a space full of possibility for fitness, it also continues to be dominated by narrow, and often dangerous, views of fitness. Everywhere we turn contradictory and confusing fitness messages abound. But the overarching theme is impossible to miss. As Louise Mansfield argues, "the emphasis on sport, fitness and leisure in late capitalism is marked by commercialization of the body..." (81). The focus on appearance and thinness (and whiteness) is obvious, a symptom of popular culture. On TV, and in pop culture more generally, fitness (for women) is first and foremost about thinness. It is about getting rid of fat, draining excess, controlling and conquering. For men, fitness is about getting bigger, harder, more cut. Fitness is programmed and promoted by celebrity personalities or star fitness gurus.

Icons from pop culture — film and music stars, Playboy bunnies, and reality–TV stars — are attached to a variety of programs and products.

Fitness can be found "On Demand" through Time Warner Cable and a variety of icons and beautiful, thin women provide everything from weight lifting workouts to burlesque for those looking to be "powerful, lean, and strong." More and more popular are infomercial fitness programs — packaged programs that provide several weeks worth of routines and some even include meal plans. Some of these, like Insanity, are extreme. Celebrities like Miley Cyrus and Reece Witherspoon are often caught by paparazzi, yoga bag slung over the shoulder, on the way to/from class. (Such a sighting was spoofed on HBO's *The Comeback*.) Well-known yogi and Hip-Hop mogul, Russell Simmons, is often the subject of yoga-related tabloid gossip; in a photo opportunity in *In Touch* magazine, Simmons can be found in seated straddle stretch, face in the sand, as his young (thin and white) girlfriend stands on his back. Celebrities' bodies are policed by the media in ways that are detrimental to all of us. As Brabazon explains, "female celebrities exercise only to maintain their svelte figure, not to become strong, fit and healthy" (65). This version of fitness certainly detracts from a holistic, transformative vision of fitness.

Even when celebrities endorse fitness that doesn't fit neatly into the confines of body image, their bodies are dragged into the conversation — most often negatively. For instance, both Oprah and Madonna have been picked apart regarding their bodies and fitness. Oprah, one of the most powerful, influential, and wealthy women in the U.S. has had to address her weight gains and losses publicly and often apologetically. She acts as a source of knowledge and inspiration on issues like body image, weight loss, and diets. And yet, body image, eating, and weight are still *an issue*. On the other end of the spectrum, Madonna is known for her devotion to yoga and to a fitness regime more generally. As she ages she is held to impossible standards and when she works out so much that the results are visible, veins bulging, she is seen as scary and extreme. "Madonna's scary arms" are discussed all over cyberspace. One article titled "What Caused Madonna's Scary Arms" sports the subtitle: "New pictures of the Material Mom reveal that no matter how much you exercise, you can't fool Father Time." The article gives a scientific analysis of how Madonna's diet and exercise regime are making her look "like a skeleton on steroids" and the author implies that all of her working out has to do with her aging (now that she's 51) and her break-up with her boyfriend. Both of these powerful women pursue fitness despite these judgments. This is one realm of celebrity fitness; others are also plagued by mainstream expectations about body size and appearance.

The kinds of "fitness" shown on programs like *The Biggest Loser, Celebrity*

Fit Club, Jackie Warner's *Intervention,* or *Dance Your Ass Off,* are the epitome of American fitness. People's lives are transformed and others are inspired, but the artificial competition puts boundaries on the transformative potential. It hurts me that people will see this version of fitness and think that it is the way to get healthy, balanced, or fit. While some people certainly want (maybe even *need*) to be yelled at and enjoy this method, and while some people need drastic interventions in their eating and lack of exercise, these shows promote unhealthy weight loss quotas and can shame those who don't lose weight quickly enough. As Tara Brabazon points out, "weight loss attracts prizes, publicity and the marketing dollar" (75). They also promote a singular vision of "fitness" and competition as integral to reaching weight loss goals. If these tactics work at all (and they do ... we can *see* the evidence), it is because they draw upon a similar American ideology — competition is healthy.[9] People's lives are transformed, but such tactics might be more challenging to maintain in the long term.

Linking fitness with products un-related to fitness is rampant throughout a variety of commercials. For instance, in a 2012 Subaru commercial we see a woman in a bike race being encouraged along by who we assume must be her husband. At first he looks concerned, like she might not make it through the race. She does, after all, look totally beat. But she keeps going and brushes away his help. He races ahead of her in their Subaru to give her encouragement along the way. He holds up signs made from cardboard and black marker, like: "You're a Machine." When she finally reaches the finish line, she looks distressed when she does not see him right away. But there he is and she looks even more distressed when he seems to be sitting there nonchalantly eating pizza. But then he opens the cover of the box and inside is the final sign of encouragement: "I love you." Like many Subaru commercials, this one paints a middle-class norm of fitness while also complicating gender stereotypes. It is the wife, not the husband, who is racing; he is her support. But, at the same time, she looks completely exhausted throughout the commercial, as if she is not really prepared for such physical exertion. But she has probably trained, and certainly hasn't eaten anything like pizza in the training process. We also get the impression that she needs this outside support to accomplish her goal. Her own strength is not enough.

Fitness has even made an appearance in beer commercials for Miller 64, a lighter-calorie beer marketed toward men who have a complicated relation-ship with fitness. From the commercials aired during the summer of 2012, it is clear that these men know that they must stay healthy and fit, if only to attract the attention of the opposite sex. It is also clear that their relationship to "the gym," and to fitness more generally, is contentious. The tagline "brewed for the better you" reminds viewers that fitness is something to be constantly worked at and even if you fall out of the cycle, you can get right back in it through attention to diet and exercise, without sacrificing "fun" or beer. The commercial states: "Returning to fitness with beer as my witness," which certainly seems to be a contradiction, but it is not, the commercial implies, because Miller 64 will be there with a fun drinking song and a montage of fit bodies, fun fitness settings, goofy shenanigans, and subterfuge fitness practices. And there are motivations for the gym as we see fit, attractive women at every turn.

In addition to being linked with beer, in popular culture yoga is connected with celebrity, with the environment, with the orient and with a variety of products most often aimed at women like tea, dog food, body wash, pain relievers, and feminine hygiene products. But yoga also makes a variety of interesting appearances on shows like FOX's *King of the Hill*. On the "Hank's Back" episode, Hank finds relief in yoga after struggling with a back injury that keeps him from his love — his job selling propane. After the medical establishment can't help him and he is forced to go on disability, Hank finds yoga and it cures him. It is clear that the practice of yoga is the remedy, not the practice of the yogi whose character embodies every stereotype and contradiction. The yoga teacher does not practice what he preaches and Hank finds his own relationship to yoga. The episode ends with him leading a yoga session at work, renaming poses to fit his interests — football and lawn care, for instance. On NBC's *Parks & Rec*, Chris is into meditation, visualization, and positive thinking as well as nutritional supplements and health concoctions. When these don't work, he turns to excessive use of therapy. While these interests are mocked through his obsession with a healthy lifestyle, meditation is portrayed as powerful when it is divorced from all the new age "frills." The hardline, "real man" boss character, Ron, is skeptical about meditation but learns the value in not thinking about anything for a period of time. Yoga has also been featured on HBO's *The Comeback* and *Dead Like Me*, and The Sundance Channel's *Girls Who Like Boys Who Like Boys*.

These T.V. representations provide some ways of critiquing more mainstream representations of fitness. Some music artists also do this through their videos that circulate widely on the internet. For instance, LMFAO's "Sexy and I Know It" has a clear satirical nature as the group members prance around in thongs, subjecting their bodies to exploitative gazes while emphasizing the unattractive attributes that thongs provide. Another parody video, "Yoga Girl" by Fog and Smog speaks to the more sexualized assumptions about yoga, exposing the ridiculousness of the stereotype (and some clever word play). And "Yoga Girls of the World" written, performed, and produced by Jocelyn

Kay Levy and Jacquelyn Richey challenge Fog and Smog by reimagining "Yoga Girl's" lyrics and images and connecting yoga practice to ways to get out into the world and make a difference. "Kanye's Workout Plan" embodies all of the sexism and misogyny that rap music is criticized for, and yet there is a parodic edge that asks us to question just exactly what all those sit ups are for. Fergie raps about fitness in her "Fergilicious" song, decked out in retro chic leotards, doing bicep curls and riding the stationary bike. Rhymefest's "One Armed Push-ups" shows the artist doing everything from smoking a cigarette to reading a book to shaving, all while doing one-armed push-ups. At the very edges of mainstream representation, the underground rap duo Dead Prez offers some potentially revolutionary advice through the song "Be Healthy" and promotes a vegetarian diet and exercise toward a healthy body and mind.[10] Visual representations of music and fitness are easily found on-line and simple searches produce an array of fitness options — some serious, some parodic, some hypnotic, and some downright ridiculous.

* * *

The influence of celebrity, business, and diet can be seen clearly in the choices for Greatist.com's previously noted "The 100 Most Influential People in Health and fitness 2012." It is no surprise that in addition to the most influential, First Lady Michelle Obama, the people on this list are visible in a number of ways. "The 100 Most Influential People in Health and Fitness 2012" argues that "there are thousands of people working every day to revolutionize the way people think about health and wellness." While eclectic and encompassing of many different aspects of health and fitness, these influencers also reflect the phenomena of "American fitness." The list is dominated by celebrity personalities, flashy brands, authoritative advice, "perfect bodies," and assumptions about what most influences health and fitness. At the margins are the goofy personalities like Richard Simmons, pushed out by sleek, sexy, serious workouts (though there are still plenty of goofy fitness instructors; we're special people that way). The trainers on this list of influencers have some connections to food through diet and weight management, and some may also be authors or inspirational leaders, but most have celebrity connections or are celebrities themselves. On this list, 34 of these most inspirational figures are trainers like Jackie Warner (#51), Jillian Michaels (#7), Tony Horton (#21, founder of P90X), "Rockin' Body," Shaun Thompson (#42), and Beto Perez (#27, founder of Zumba). The celebrity connection with personal trainers is a key to the ways in which we understand mainstream American fitness. We idolize the hard bodies and svelte figures of our celebrities, and so it makes sense that we might look to celebrity trainers for workout tips and guidance. And in some cases trainers and celebrities work closely to market a particular workout.

LL Cool J's Platinum Workout not only illustrates this celebrity connection, it also illustrates some of the patriarchal (if not also sexist) ideals and assumptions of American fitness. LL Cool J is not only known for his physique, he is also known for his sensitive rap lyrics like his 1987 hit, "I Need Love," a song considered a major "panty dropper" by many women of my generation. LL Cool J is a sex symbol and he has the body that everyone wants. He argues that **"there is nothing inherently unique about my body"**; what is unique is the **"revolutionary workout system"** (xii, original emphasis) that he and "Scooter" created. While the authors of this book are LL Cool J (James Todd Smith) and Dave "Scooter" Honig (his trainer) with Jeff O'Connell (executive writer for *Men's Health* magazine), it is LL Cool J's voice we hear loud and clear. It is his literal and figurative image that sells the workout. He motivates his reader through his personal impetus and workout journey, explaining that after he made the film *Rollerball* he decided he had to get serious about his body and "take it to the next level"; he writes, "I achieved that, and it changed my life, both physically and emotionally" (xi). He wants the reader to change their life too, to experience the "enlightenment" and the "paradigm shift" (xi); his Platinum Workout, he argues, is the way to do this. And the workout offered in this glossy book is certainly an effective workout, as is any other workout. All fitness pursuits take time, discipline, consistency, knowledge, adaptation, and work. But the specifics of the Platinum Workout are an interesting example of gender and "American fitness."

While the book makes several attempts to reach out to women, the bulk of the book is clearly targeting men. For instance, in the tips and information section references are made to testosterone and male growth hormone. The inclusion of a female model might seem to be inclusive toward women but since she is the only figure who appears without a name or a voice, it seems more likely that her toned body and short shorts are eye candy as much as an attempt toward inclusion. Even so, LL Cool J writes, "Scooter and I both feel strongly that women should train like men, and vice versa" (210). And while he cites some research that backs this fact, neither "like men" nor "vice versa" are defined; however, the assumption is the Platinum Workout is the way in which men train. But, he offers the "Diamond Body" and the opportunity to get "cut and sparkling" (210) for "emergency" use like a wedding or when "the time comes to slip into last year's bikini" (211). This Diamond Workout emphasizes the "butt, hamstrings, and other body parts that we know you want to firm up" (211). But women "shouldn't waste a second worrying about morphing into a muscle man" (210). All of these sexist assumptions are not unusual in the world of mainstream American fitness. However, it gets worse before it gets better. LL Cool J quells the ladies' worries about bulking up by adding "(Believe me, ladies, I want to be the hardest thing in the bed.)" (210). He then reminds us how the "Ladies Love Cool James" and assures us that "you'll really love me when you're walking down the aisle in your wedding dress looking your best ever" (211). And while this certainly fits the expectations of some women's exercise goals, it gets a bit creepy when he writes: "light some candles when you work out, feel good about yourself, and then buy yourself some flowers at the end of the week, baby. Sign my name on the card. Oh, and get a massage" (211). Elsewhere he speaks to the importance of massage as recovery, but here it sounds like a sex-charged luxury. If the suggestions weren't ridiculous, then the tone would certainly speak for itself.

Throughout the workout such comments continue with a condescending tone like: "we really zero in on your quads, hamstrings, and glutes — exactly what women love to focus on. You're not worried about having 18-inch biceps, but you do want tight hips, glutes, and hamstrings. Am I right?" (212). Right or not, women's worries and desires concerning their bodies cannot be so neatly encapsulated, nor so detached from the source of our anxieties (like men who have such expectations for or about us). Even sound advice is undercut in this way such as: "a complete woman needs a complete body, and that includes stretching" (213). Elsewhere stretching is emphasized as an important component of a total body fitness regime. In fact the "Bend So You Don't Break" chapter emphasizes this idea and includes photos illustrating the stretches — all performed by the female model, not LLCool J.

Advice is also offered for those who may not be supportive of your new body, advice that is "especially relevant to the ladies" (224). LL Cool J makes a direct attempt to intervene in domestic violence as he argues that jealous men might attempt to make us feel bad and notes that "if that goes down, that's not where you need to be" (224). While the scenario is certainly possible, the paternalistic quality exudes the patriarchal assumption about the need to protect women, even women who have gained self-confidence and physical strength. Finally, while there are many aspects of the overall book that deal with nutrition, food choices, and discipline, "one final word" before the breakdown of the workouts addresses the "need to follow the platinum diets closely.... Don't succumb to eating food you shouldn't because you're in search of instant gratification. Maybe you're depressed, so you want to curl up with a cupcake and watch a movie. Or whisper sweet nothings to a half gallon of ice cream. Making sweet love to those banana muffins" (213). The final line would have sufficed: "You can't use food as a source of comfort. You've got to eat to live, not live to eat" (213). While all of this might be important advice, the ways in which the "general" audience of men is addressed (even as it assumes inclusion of women) is quite different from the ways in which this same advice is delivered to women directly.

* * *

In all of these pop culture (mis-)representations, there are also some potentially transformative moments. When First lady Michelle Obama appeared on Chef Robert Irvine's show, *Restaurant: Impossible*, just one of her many television appearances, she brought a national campaign to a make-over show. In addition to challenging Chef Irvine to make over a community center for the non-profit group, Horton's Kids, in Washington D.C., the show highlights the projects that Michelle Obama has been a part of like the organic garden at the White House, linking fitness and food. Chef Irvine points out that she is "one of the fittest first ladies" ever, and in many ways Michelle Obama has become an icon of fitness, promoting yoga at the annual Easter Egg Roll through a "Yoga Garden with colorful mats and helpful teachers" (Broad 2). On a spoof of Republicans on TV show, *30 Rock*, Liz Lemon's conservative boss, Jack, attempts to lure ultra-conservatives to contribute to his Super Pac by promoting Republican gossip, including the charge that Michelle Obama is on steroids.[11] The comment is meant to be kryptonite to Liz Lemon's liberal feminism. Michelle is a force in and out of popular culture.

Michelle Obama has also teamed up with Beyoncé to create a fitness dance routine for Let's Move! Beyoncé's "Move Your Body" is a remix of her song "Get Me Bodied," which has quite a different message and purpose. And yet, it is easily adaptable, including fitness moves and dance moves, and delivered with the signature style of the diva. It is both instructional and performative. While the song is not available on Amazon.com or iTunes, the music video and variations can be found on YouTube. The official video includes Beyoncé dancing in a school cafeteria with kids; she's decked out in her typical revealing fashion right down to her high heels, the biggest travesty to this example of fitness. She can work it in heels after years of practice, but what kind of message is she sending about fitness or about fit women? Feminized fashion clearly trumps the fitness element. The controversy surrounding her refusal to walk in high heels in the cold after rehearsing for her performance at President Obama's inauguration (the secret service allowed a car to come pick her and Jay-Z up instead) seems to undercut this version of fitness.[12] "Move Your Body" has succeeded in getting us to move our bodies, but it will not allow us to move our minds too far away from mainstream expectations. Challenging mainstream pop culture takes more critical movement.

Fitness Fads and Gadgets

"Every year, buzzwords and new fads keeping popping up to fool many people into thinking that they need this or that to reach their goals. Words like core, functional, tone, dynamic etc. are used and abused to confuse people. The fitness industry continues to make money by keeping people confused and result-less. That way it can continue to market its fads by using buzzwords and catch phrases."
— Libby Wescombe, "Oh Fitness Industry,
Where Art Thou Balance?"

Gina Kolata notes that the late seventies was the start of "a new era of fitness promotion" (48). Running became a popular fitness pastime, with people who identified themselves as runners increasing from 100,000 people in the early sixties to 30 million by the late seventies. "Women took aerobics classes," she notes, "their popularity boosted by Jane Fonda" (48). When Jack LaLanne opened his gym in Oakland in 1936, Kolata notes, "athletes had to sneak in" (226). It wasn't until Arnold Schwarzenegger in the 1970s that "weight lifting became acceptable" and provided "an impetus for ordinary people to decide to lift weights" (225).[13] Nike and Reebok became major players and an entire industry rose to the challenge of not simply supplying the needed goods and services but creating an industry that produces goods and services that make us think we need such *things* to be fit.

The commercial nature of fitness centers and the fitness industry is a by-product of our consumer culture — the gadgets and constant "innovations" and the desire to always develop new forms, new products, new "better" versions of the same. Certainly some of these innovations are important and are not simply servants to the capitalist master. And certainly anything that inspires people to move their bodies can't be all bad. But this approach to fitness will inevitably fail in the long run. If we think about fitness as something that needs to be constantly stoked with new stimulus, then we forget that fitness comes from the inside out as well as the outside in. We forget that fitness is something to be crafted and maintained. Further, as Jaana Parviainen argues, "the costs of new product/service development in the global market have risen to also prohibit the emergence of new brands" (50). Even the best ideas may not make it to the status of fad in this global market, let alone have the opportunity to develop staying power. If fitness cannot be marketed widely, it cannot be accessed in masse, let alone locally.

Some of the gyms where I've taught have valued the almost constant influx of new equipment or new, trendy programs. Others have had barely any equipment at all — rows of dented, dinged, and dusty hand weights and steps. Or less. Some fitness centers or gyms operate under the assumption that new equipment and new gadgets will bring in new participants and new revenue. Sometimes this is true. Manufactured fitness programs like BTS can increase participation and, at least in theory, attract new members.[14] The strategic branding of Zumba makes it more popular than classes that are much better, safer workouts. But, overwhelmingly, fads are just that and the only real way to get new members or new participants is to keep them through quality fitness programs and personal connections. A shiny apparatus or a mass-marketing deluge is not going to keep someone in the workout mode — a shift in consciousness will. When people understand and experience the benefits of regular exercise, they will come and they will stay. But many fitness centers struggle with how to get people in the doors.

Following the "extreme" trends of recreation often portrayed in popular culture, fitness has developed more "hardcore" fitness programs like Cross-Fit and Beachbody's P90X. These high-intensity interval training programs (HIIT), like Tabata (of Japanese origins), are the latest trend in fitness, even though their recent incarnations are not really very new and certainly aren't all that revolutionary. While CrossFit claims adaptability across special populations ("perfect application for any committed individual regard-less of experience" from "elderly individuals with heart disease and cage fighters one month out from televised bouts"), it is clearly targeted for, and sold as, "the principal strength and conditioning program for many police academies and tactical operations teams, military special operations units, champion martial artists, and hundreds of other elite and professional ath-letes worldwide." It is raw, often practiced in garages or minimalist spaces. The appeal of this program is based upon our associations of fitness with athletes and military personnel, similar to the appeal of Kenneth Cooper's Air Force–derived point system. CrossFit specializes in not specializing, not letting the body get comfortable in a particular routine. They claim that "the needs of Olympic athletes and our grandparents differ by degree not kind. Our terrorist hunters, skiers, mountain bike riders and housewives have found their best fitness from the same regimen." A very similar program, P90X, on the other hand, markets itself as "extreme" as it uses "muscle confusion" to train the body. This program also speaks to un-gendered expectations as it includes and encourages women to build strength and do the full exercises instead of modifications.[15] When Presidential candidate, Mitt Romney, announced his choice for vice presidential running mate, Paul Ryan, one sell-ing point the media focused on was Ryan's physical fitness, credited to his P90X workouts.

Perhaps even more "extreme" is Insanity, "the hardest workout ever put on DVD."[16] The Insanity website promises "a year's worth of results in just

60 days." Beachbody fitness personality, Shaun T (full name Shaun Thompson and also of Hip Hop Abs fame) is considered by some Insanity participants as a personal trainer; it's not just a DVD exercise program, we're urged to believe. Shaun T describes Insanity as "a shortcut to the body you want" and tells potential consumers: "I think you're crazy not to try Insanity." The site plays on the idea of "insanity" in multiple iterations including the claim that Insanity will help you gain confidence (stated while images of skydiving fill the screen). The voice over on the introductory video argues that "insanity is extremely hard but that doesn't mean it's crazy." And Insanity appeals not only to the potential customer's desire to embrace an "insane" approach to working out; it also appeals to the average American's laziness and desire to get results fast and easily. Convenient: "You don't need to drag yourself to the gym day after day. Step out of bed, you're in the gym." Efficient: "use your body to transform your body." Easy: "only 40 minutes a day."

And Insanity, in its self promotion, cannot help but associate itself with the military, not only in its bootcamp stylings, but also in its testimonials. One testimonial includes a woman who purchased Insanity while her husband was deployed. She says, "I knew that I needed to change something about myself. And I knew that I wanted to be a hot wife when my husband got back from Afghanistan." While there are many ways in which we might interpret the first part of her statement — her desire to change something about herself— in multiple ways, her second desire is immediately identifiable with mainstream American fitness ideology. The woman further explains that she "ordered it reluctantly and then threw up on the first day." This comment is spliced and followed by Shaun T saying to his Insanity participants, "that's what I want from you...." Ultimately, Insanity is credited with providing the means to a "new lifestyle I can share with my husband," reinforcing not only the extreme results of the Insanity program but also the institutions of military and marriage, and by extension, patriarchy.[17] Capitalism is also entwined as the program costs 3 monthly payments of 39.95 (plus 24.95 shipping and handling); the price is ambiguous since the site promises "a year's worth of results in just 60 days."

One thing that many of these fads and gadgets have in common is the infomercial — proliferating late-night television as well as the internet. This fitness form merges business acumen with flashy commercial appeal and easy promises. Zumba's popularity can be directly linked with the visibility of their infomercial. Les Mills can reach outside of health clubs, marketing their Body Pump program on DVD as "Les Mills Pump." Through Beachbody there are a plethora of programs, many of which are steeped in masculinity and buff possibilities: 10 Minute Trainer, Tapout XT (with a wrestling theme),

Insanity, Brazil Butt Lift, Turbofire, and a bodybuilding program—Body Beast—which encourages us to "man up" and boasts that one can "get big. And get noticed" by going "from scrawny to brawny" in just "90 days or less." The audience is clear through the diet: "don't expect some wimpy lettuce wedge diet. Be prepared to eat like never before, and then eat some more. Get ready to EAT LIKE A MAN." A feminine version is offered through "Metamorphosis" by Tracey Anderson which is touted as "organic plastic surgery" and a "body reshaping system." Even supplements have their own commercials and infomercials. TruBiotics claims "we know what it takes to look good on the outside" even though their product is for intestinal health. A flashy, glitzy commercial (more music video than infomercial) for Xenadrine offers an "extreme" approach to weight loss, akin to the extreme claims of Insanity and P90X. It claims to be a product for "weight loss revolution" as slim, toned bodies fill the screen.

The popular media texts combine with the power of the market so that "such ideas about the exercising body provide seeds for an entire fitness lifestyle through which continued consumption of the fitness industry becomes possible" (Kennedy and Markula 4). The lifestyle promoted by the fads and gadgets, icons and representations, is one that requires constant consumption. It requires innovation rather than introspection, trust of an industry rather than instinct. As Jaana Parviainen argues, "to create an attractive fitness brand, a company does not necessarily need innovative products/services but something or someone with a personality that gives vitality to the brand" (51). Thus, Zumba and P90X may not be the best forms of exercise, but they are promoted by the best-known fitness personalities. This is a larger American reality— the endorsement and marketing might just overwhelm the worth of the product itself at the same time that worthy products never make their ways onto our televisions or our shelves, let alone our lives.

Institutionalized Fitness

"Aerobics has a special status as the McDonalds of sport: cheap, accessible and fast. In one hour, every muscle in the body is worked and moved.... It is also a customised [sic] practice, with diverse sessions attracting distinct cliental. Aerobics is a salad bar of opportunities and choices."
— Tara Brabazon, "Fitness Is a Feminist Issue" (66)[18]

"The industry is still too fixated on fads instead of classic movement forms. It's still hung up on instant weight loss, at the expense of permanent weight loss. It's overly infatuated with how people look, rather than how they feel. It still causes too many injuries. It's still too regi-

mented. It's still too boring. It's still too macho and masculine. And
it's really never gotten past the idea that pain is necessary."
— Debbie Rosas and Carlos Rosas, *The Nia Technique* (24)

Fitness is an unregulated industry — a competitive system of certification
programs and an increasing number of specialized training programs, uneven
in quality, preparation, price, and value. Fitness is sold to potential instructors
and practitioners as a set of skills, but, more often, provide a set of knowledge.
Some trainings offer in-depth, hands-on instruction, some require participants
to pass a test in order to be certified. Some programs require a monthly membership fee; some provide new choreography periodically. Some certification
programs require only a test, taken on a computer. Some require extensive
study and practical application is also tested or reviewed. Some training programs are housed within universities or private gyms. Some are provided by
businesses devoted to developing fitness programs. Some are one day or less;
some take years. With such a wide variety of possible practitioners, trainers,
certifications and types of programs, deciding which fitness path to pursue —
as an instructor, let alone as a participant — can be quite overwhelming. Gina
Kolata relates some of the incongruence and irony of fitness certifications
through her daughter's pursuit of a personal training certification. "It turned
out to be easy — all she had to do was take and pass a written exam. She did
not have to show she knew her way around a weight room or that she knew
how to run or how to use an elliptical trainer. She did not have to see a single
client, nor did she even have to set foot in a gym. But she did have to pay"
(241). Ultimately, Kolata argues my point: "certification is a business" (245).

Because my training was a university class for credit and included academic preparation as well as hands-on practical training (however limited this
practical training was), I never went through a formal certification program.
I have never had a problem getting a job. I ended up teaching not only fitness
classes but fitness instructor training classes and mentoring other instructors
through a "shadow" apprentice training. I developed my own approaches and
curriculum in both cases. I felt that this kind of training was organic; it
required an understanding of the building blocks for teaching fitness and
assured that instructors were committed and motivated. To teach from this
basis of training is to constantly create and re-create fitness routines. It requires
creativity, close observation, memorization, planning ahead, and adapting
what doesn't work. This is what I love about fitness, but it is certainly not
the norm in American fitness, which has become standardized even as it is
largely unregulated.[19]

Standardization means that fitness is consistent, transferable, exportable,
sellable, marketable, and trademarkable. These fitness brands are successful

when the "interface" of the brand is not just in one space but across the internet, clothing products, DVDs, and in face-to-face classes, as Jaana Parviainen argues. Ironically, fitness has learned from the trends in the fast food industry described by Eric Schlosser in his muckraking book, *Fast Food Nation*. He argues that "every facet of American life has now been franchised or chained" and "the key to a successful franchise ... can be expressed in one word: 'uniformity'" (5). Both certifications and fitness training programs are for-profit business ventures that often care less about the quality of instructors they are churning out and more about the brand of their fitness product. For instance, to become a "Flirty Girl Fitness Instructor" you can "attend a one-day Flirtification workshop or complete the At-Home Flirtification course." Their full-page advertisement in *IDEA Fitness Journal* might appeal to instructors who already have a skill set and are looking to pay $200 for new choreography. But such skills aren't a prerequisite. With "everything you need to get started" you can "dance today, teach tomorrow."

Like food, fitness has direct impacts on people's lives and bodies. Both lose nutritional value through standardization. In his book, *The Science of Yoga*, this unregulated nature of the yoga industry is one of William J. Broad's biggest criticisms. Even as he recognizes the limitations of science, he looks to science to not only help us understand the ways in which yoga can contribute to our health, fitness, and well-being, but also the ways in which it might regulate this "bustling industry" (218). But Broad seeks more regulation. "It's not like a religion or modern medicine," he writes, "where rigorous schooling, licensing, and boards seek to produce a high degree of conformity. And forget about government oversight" (4). Do we really want our yoga to be more like a religion or a medical science? Is conformity really the answer to what American yoga (or fitness more generally) *should* look like? He takes it as an "encouraging sign ... that government authorities in the United States and elsewhere have started to fund the science of yoga..." (219). Others might visualize red tape, diverted funds, pet projects, overspending, corrupt agendas, and other associations we might have with "government authorities."

While Broad's point is an important one, his study of yoga is far from the "impartial evaluation" (9) he claims it to be. The fault is not with Broad here but, rather, with our Western notions of objectivity and our value of governmental oversight. As Jaana Parviainen argues, over the past 15 years, "pre-choreographed fitness programs, licenses, trademarks and brands..." have been used in part toward guaranteeing quality. "Fitness classes, in particular standardized and pre-choreographed fitness programs like Les Mills, are largely predictable, pre-selected, and highly circumscribed" (53). Parviainen argues "that the license-based fitness work has actually deadened rather than empowered professional instructors' scope for action in fitness industry" (56). Such programs certainly limit creativity, adaptability, inspiration, connection, and the ways in which an instructor interfaces with her participants. Some people just don't like these standardized programs and others prefer them to classes that are designed by individual instructors. After accompanying a colleague to a Zumba class Pirkko Markula writes in her *Psychology Today* blog, "To my surprise I did not enjoy the class and feel almost *guilty*. What is wrong with me when I cannot join the fun of dancing?" But she also concludes that she is "not alone with [her] ambivalent feelings" and considers Parviainen's research about Les Mills programs. "Parviainen concludes," Markula argues, "rather negatively, that standardized exercise classes are characterized by imitation, impersonal co-motion, and interpassivity instead of interactivity." Manufactured fitness proscribes loyalty to the "brand" and the unique aspects of its particular program, which can limit instructor's freedom. Thus, manufactured fitness also limits "scope for action" and the ability to influence industry transformation is worth further exploration.[20]

* * *

For a long time I adamantly rejected manufactured fitness programs like the Les Mills series. I found, and still find, many of these classes to be dangerous — weight classes that encourage participants to use too much weight with too-fast repetitions, yoga fusion classes that rarely hold a pose for more than a few seconds. These programs create choreography and then package it. The instructors memorize the routines and teach the same routine for several months. Every class has the same structure, the same songs, the same moves and while instructors bring some aspect of personality and can sometimes change things up, the purpose of these classes is that someone can go to a class and know exactly what to expect. And when I have witnessed or experienced such fitness classes, I have thought to myself, *how horrible*. As an instructor, this means death. This approach takes almost everything I love about teaching fitness and extracts it from the process. The online discussions surrounding the infamous split between Les Mills and BTS are enlightening in terms of understanding the strengths and weaknesses of both programs as well as the tension between manufactured fitness and "free-style" fitness programs and approaches. Ultimately, the discussion goes back and forth between the various aspects of fitness programs: music, choreography, philosophy, trainers, and other details. Some instructors are loyal to Les Mills, others to BTS. Finally, toward the end of this conversation, a few instructors critique the very base of this discussion. Why should we be forced to choose between these two similar programs? They are simply versions of the same thing. Whatever happened to "freestyle" fitness instruction where the instructor has free reign over music, choreography, and tone and more limited control over space, participants, and time?[21]

Despite my principled and practical aversion to manufactured fitness, I fell in love with the BTS program, Group Groove, as a participant. I began to crave the predictability and to savor the ability to burn the routines into my mind and body. I crave the movements. Recently I became a Group Groove instructor. I never planned to take any manufactured fitness trainings. I have no desire to spend time memorizing someone else's choreography, someone else's music choices, according to someone else's time schedule. I have no desire to take a training focused specifically on the teaching of one kind of class and then creating a video to prove that I have mastered their style and skill set. I will continue to create fitness organically, but I now have an appreciation for some of these classes, some of the styles, and some of their purposes. I love Group Groove and I love teaching it. Group Groove is my guilty pleasure. I "stomp, wiggle, jiggle, hip hop, shimmy, shake, glide" in this "dynamic fusion of dance styles [that] creates an all out cardio jam designed to be the coolest way to get fit." The mission to "get more people moving" is an admirable one; the cheesy description is only the marketing side of this program. The quality is in the class structure and choreography, and in the results of the workout — increased stamina, agility, and speed. The trade offs are worth it.

While industry regulation is not a bad idea in theory, the reality of current regulation is a joke. The flaws are ultimately the result of more regulated fitness programs and a shrinking of "freestyle" instructors whose knowledge is multi-layered, practical, informed, experiential, and creative. Such skills are qualities that cannot be fully developed in a few hours of training; they can't be easily measured or mandated. The most problematic regulation comes through certification bodies like ACE, AFAA, and ACSM.[22] While these certifying bodies perform a range of important services like continuing education oversight and informal opportunities for education through e-mail updates and the *IDEA Fitness Journal*, for instance, in my experience, such a certification has been utterly inconsequential (outside the drain on my bank account). After about 10 years of teaching in the fitness industry with plenty of trainings but without any certifications, I decided to pay the money to ACE and take the group fitness certification test. It would, in theory, make me more money. (In reality, it has not.) I would be moving across the country and some gyms required the certification. Despite the fact that I had been employed continuously as a fitness instructor for over a decade, even after moving several times, I thought maybe it wouldn't be a bad idea to be certified. Over $350 later I took a test on a computer that asked me a variety of questions, most of which had nothing to do with what I do day-to-day, class-to-class as a group fitness instructor. Most were full of scientific jargon and concerned minute details related to health problems that were not a part of the scope of my work. I passed the computer test, without distinction and below my high standards, and was awarded a certification that would expire 2 years later.

I had two years to accumulate 2.0 continuing education credits from programs approved by ACE, partnered with ACE. In the midst of a new job and three moves in two years, I did not accumulate any credits. And yet, my knowledge and experience with fitness grew. I began teaching belly dancing and choreographing dozens of new songs. I took new classes and learned from other instructors and from on-line videos. But I did not accumulate the required credits. The yoga training that I planned to take would only count toward 1.4 CECs. With .6 other necessary credits, and with more than $100 necessary to recertify, I decided to let my certification lapse. I felt strapped into a system that exists not to supplement or augment my skills and knowledge, not to better my teaching, but to contain and control me. They take my money, offering only rules and regulations, trends and tests. They decide what programs are appropriate to my fitness career, let alone my fitness life. As helpful as *IDEA Fitness Journal* has been, my ACE certification is not worth the costs. And yet, the time may come when I have to recertify in order to continue to do what I love.

Not every program that offers fitness training, choreography, knowledge, routines, or products qualify as "manufactured"; many have value, perhaps even revolutionary potential. And a more regulated industry is not necessarily the answer. Instead, critical vigilance is a must. Feminist and cultural critic, bell hooks, describes the role of the "enlightened witness" who must be "critically vigilant." In this role we can, hooks argues, "both resist certain kinds of conservatizing representation and at the same time create new and exciting representations" (*Cultural Criticism*). This figure holds accountable those in positions of power and influence; in the case of fitness, we must be sure that the superficial or economic benefits of fitness do not outweigh the deeper meanings of fitness. The instructor is ultimately responsible for applying fitness knowledge and the tools we gain through training are the foundation. This foundation is in need of repair and the system for building needs to be restructured. Those of us with experience are responsible for mentoring and supporting new instructors. We might also take responsibility for supporting skill-based training instead of brand-based training. Such skills give manufactured fitness its ultimate value. The best programs are delivered by skilled, experienced instructors and created by conscious, critical instructors/programs. This work is, in part, embedded in our expectations for health, sport, and science. It is worked out by transformative innovators.

Sketches: Transformative Innovators: Complicating "Cardio" and Democratizing Yoga

Throughout all of my sketches, and throughout this work as a whole, I pay tribute to transformative innovators — women (and some men) who have transformed themselves, who work every day to transform the lives of others. Instructors who innovate on what they have been taught in order to create a dynamic, energetic, organic workout for their participants. Participants who adapt movements and adopt new dimensions of their personalities when they dance, shake, shimmy, step, kick, or strut. Some of these dynamic innovators find their inspiration, in part, in the teachings and trainings of other dynamic innovators.

The "transformative innovators" I feature here have built a foundation for others to enhance their fitness lives, to seek education and training, to serve communities. These are only a handful of such people and the kinds of work that they do requires constant innovation rooted in traditions of practice. These brief sketches represent countless other innovative, grounded, hard-working, devoted individuals. This an homage to those who have inspired me and whose work continues to inspire countless others.

Beth Shaw: YogaFit Training Systems

"Business without a greater purpose, a purpose beyond profit, has no point."

— Beth Shaw

Beth Shaw is the founder and President of a fitness business that works — YogaFit Training Systems, Inc. She works with a team of dynamic, committed individuals who have expanded, and continue to build YogaFit, which integrates almost every aspect of yoga into its business model: a teacher-training program; a provider of instructional DVDs, music collections on CD, apparel and merchandise; and innovation of yoga in a fitness context. But Beth's business model is one of responsibility. She writes, "I've always felt that no matter how big or small your business is, it is important to give back. How rich or poor you feel is all relative, and we all have the power to make a positive difference on this planet in some way" (xii). Toward these beliefs, YogaFit encourages its instructors to give back through required community service hours to complete the level one training and Beth Shaw models this service through her work as an animal rights activist and her nonprofit organization, Visionary Women in Fitness (276). Shaw has a business philosophy that melds well with the lessons of yoga while it also has the ability to be a successful business model in a cut-throat capitalist system. As Dr. William Kent Larkin argues in his foreword to *Beth Shaw's YogaFit*, Beth "has developed a program of integrated methodologies that makes yoga accessible to everyone" (vii).

He continues, "what Beth has done is build a model that is for everybody, that is applicable, that works, and that lasts over time.... You are not molded into a program; YogaFit is molded and formed for you" (vi). This is, in fact, one of the underlying principles of the YogaFit essence: "feeling and listening to your body" (14). *Beth Shaw's YogaFit* outlines the particular YogaFit principles as well as providing an accessible guide to practicing yoga, complete with a breakdown of "purposeful poses." This book is yet another tool to bring yoga to the masses, but YogaFit goes much further and deeper than this book. For teachers of yoga, YogaFit's training system offers an extensive set of general and specialized yoga teacher trainings. The base of trainings, level one through five, provide a foundation for yoga teachers as well as the foundation toward certification through Yoga Alliance, the national certification organization. An array of other trainings covering topics like anatomy, modifications, props, breathing, weight management, and special populations complete the certification. "YogaFit has trained more that 75,000 fitness instructors in six continents" (276) and it continues to grow, most recently developing a yoga therapy program.

As YogaFit continues to expand its business and programs, it stays true to its roots in the idea of "yoga for the masses." The YogaFit "Essence" highlights the mind/body approach of yoga, emphasizing: "breathing, feeling and listening to your body, letting go of expectations, letting go of competition, letting go of judgment, and staying in the present moment" (14). It's 2012–13 facelift to its website speaks to this desire to reach people and demystify the practice of yoga (while not losing its mystic quality). This American form of yoga is layered, hybrid, and accessible.

Debbie Rosas and Carlos AyaRosas: The Nia Technique

These dynamic personalities credit the industry's turn to, and attention to mind/body practices of fitness, to their development of Nia. In their book,

The Nia Technique, they argue that "these days, there's nothing strange to most sophisticated people about the concepts of mind-body fitness or cross-training or getting fit with healing arts..." (20). These are the foundations of contemporary mind/body fitness, "inaugurated" through Nia, as Debbie and Carlos argue. Nia certainly is a revolutionary form of fitness, one that encourages "The Body's Way" and pleasure rather than pain. The technique is done with bare feet and an incorporation of emotion and playfulness. It is "whole-being fitness" (17). It became a "nationwide phenomenon during the 1990s" (23) and is practiced around the world as well. While Carlos retired after 2010, Debbie continues to teach Nia and to grow the program, offering "the new face of Nia." According to Nia teacher and trainer, Sophie Marsh, "taking off the mask to be wholly in truth, letting go of how things had been done before, and opening to a collective creativity, knowledge and wisdom is *the new face of Nia.*"

Jaana Parviainen details a similar approach to fitness in the work of Marja Putkisto who developed her own version of a mind/body approach to fitness (what Parviainen refers to as "slow movement"), the Method Pukisto, which grew during the 1990s and has recently become more popular in the U.K. and Finland. "She 'listens' to her body and her body tells her how to proceed healing herself and developing tools for well-being" (48). Her methods were not immediately recognized by the "fitness world" which was "concentrated on celebrating aerobics 'to feel the burn'" (48). These are the same industry trends that drove Debbie and Carlos to develop a non-impact aerobics. Nia evolved as a result of the weaknesses that Debbie and Carlos found in their bodies, representing the weaknesses in the fitness industry. The development of Nia speaks to an evolution of Nia as well as to fitness. Debbie and Carlos tell this story in *The Nia Technique.*

This book also provides a dense set of tools — including philosophies, breakdown of the movements, deep descriptions of the related anatomy and physiology, workouts/cycles, and a Nia Workout Menu of foci — for those who might want to practice Nia on their own. A few DVDs are also available for such practice and people can search for Nia instructors on Nia's website. This book provides thoughtful, helpful advice for finding a more empowered, conscious fitness; they are ideas that are worth "stepping into."[23] For me, the most important fundamental of Nia speaks to its powerful vision of fitness: "*The Joy of Movement Is the Secret of Fitness.* Stop exercising. Start moving. Follow the pleasure principle: If it feels good, do it; if it doesn't, stop" (16; authors' emphasis). This is advice that I have built into my own fitness practice and philosophy of teaching. Such ideas turn "no pain, no gain" on its head and offers a more fitting fitness approach than most popular understandings.

One of the most powerful things about *The Nia Technique* is its weaving of testimonials throughout the narrative and instruction. Such testimonials can also be found on the NiaNow website as well as on the webpages of individual instructors. The testimonials speak about being touched by, connected to, even healed by Nia. And I have experienced this myself. Nia can be a magical kind of fitness experience if we let it. The New-Agey-ness, the unfamiliarity, the freedom of Nia, can all be intimidating and if Nia suffers from anything it is a lack of understanding from a fitness industry that has a different set of values and a public that has been saturated in these different values. However, Debbie and Carlos are right. Nia is like chocolate. "You can't describe it — you have to taste it" (3). And while there are some people who don't like chocolate, those who like it, love it and can't live without it.

Fitness Affiliations: Health, Sport, and Science

"I want to win as an athlete and shine as a woman."
— Natalie Coughlin, Olympic swimmer in a Pantene commercial

"The Sport of Fitness Has Arrived."
— Reebok ad campaign

"The simplest definition of a sport is that which involves men and balls. When one or both of these variables are removed, the determination of a sport becomes more tenuous. Aerobics includes few men and no balls, so claiming a sporting definition is difficult."
— Tara Brabazon, "Fitness Is a Feminist Issue" (66)

While fitness is its own concept, distinct from health and with different ways and means than sport, both health and sport are a part of fitness. Science is often the link between health and fitness and sport and fitness, measuring the impacts — positive and negative — on the human body, and less often the human mind. For instance, early developments in fitness research by Dr. Kenneth Cooper were intimately linked to health and yet the field of health is also distinctly separate from that of fitness. Likewise, sport is certainly measurable according to a particular set of rules and expectations. There are winners and losers and we might assume that the winners are more fit competitors in their sport (or that they are taking performance enhancers). Though our assumptions of fitness are often based on physical performance, a fitness of mind — the ability to perform under pressure — is equally important in the realm of sports. While aspects of sports and health are measurable, the concept and state of fitness are far less quantifiable.

Health, like fitness, is difficult to quantify. What is healthy for one person may not be so for another person. But health (setting aside appearance) is certainly our primary reason for exercising. And "fitness" assumes a level of health. The Greatist.com "influencers" are also instructive here. On this list, 21 people were involved almost exclusively in the medical aspects of health and fitness. Some of these were also connected to food, and a few were also celebrities, but the majority were doctors — clear examples of people who provide ultimate authority through medical expertise. Some are celebrities like #48, TV host, Dr. Travis Stork. A couple of these medical experts embraced alternative medicine like #50, Chris Kresser, who "quickly earned a large following interested in dissecting health and wellness information and learning how to live healthier, more empowered lives." The influence of medical opinions is often cited, and the science behind fitness holds even more weight when it is backed by medical science and the authority of doctors.

With the weight of authority, science has been a primary vehicle for understanding fitness. As William Broad writes in his study of the science of yoga, "The guidelines for aerobic exercise developed slowly over the course of the twentieth century.... Ultimately, the enterprise drew on the work of hundreds of scientists" (75). Academia provides a wide variety of avenues to explore the science of fitness as do government grants. Whether studying aerobic exercise or strength training, lung capacity or caloric expenditure, science can measure at least some of the results of fitness. And here there is much overlap with health and sports. Further, sports, health, and science are three fields that have been historically dominated by men. Thus, their approaches are masculine as the norm and even though women have made plenty of important contributions to these fields, men still dominate them. This dominance, as well as the congruent dominance of men in exercise and sport science settings, and the continued dominance of men in institutional positions of power related to fitness, has also influenced the ways in which we understand women's exercise. Some feminist researchers "see exercise as a feminizing activity that supports the oppressive ideology of masculinity which assigns women as polar opposites and thus, inferior to men" (Kennedy and Markula 9). Since sports, health, and science rely on this polarization to some extent, women's inferiority is transferable across these forms, which bleeds over into their relation to fitness.

Health and sport are perhaps less connected than health and fitness or sport and fitness, but health and sport are structurally similar. Both assume a rigid structure of rules. Science assumes objectivity and uses measurement. The American Medical Association has strict guidelines that determine the state of one's cardiovascular health for instance, even if one's overall picture of health might be more difficult to measure. In sport, the rulebook is enforced and interpreted through authority figures — the referee or umpire has the last judgment. This is one place where fitness differs. While there are plenty of rules that govern fitness, there is also a freedom to fitness that can manifest in very different ways than in sports, through the mind and body. As we engage in intuitive movement — our way of moving with or without structure — we strengthen the mind/body connection and engage the creative and critical modes. And this is one of the dangerous realms of fitness — that which is not quantifiable. We value what science can tell us about our bodies, about our health and fitness; science is an authority. We trust science.

Gina Kolata explores science but is not limited simply to what science can tell us about the subject of fitness. She also looks at the ways in which science relates to mythologies of exercise: "I'm a skeptic," she writes, "conditioned by long years of science reporting" (9). For instance, while science has much to tell us about how much weight to lift, how many repetitions to do, and how to build muscle, "most of us simply assume that if we start to work our muscles, something will happen — our bodies will change in shape and maybe size" (233). Further, as one of her sources notes, "many who lift weights actually resist learning what science has to say" (236). With weight training, "'It's got its own culture'" (236) and the ways in which people work out is directly tied to the ways in which such fitness pursuits are marketed. The "new programs" that fill the pages of magazines, DVDs, and websites are only variations on a long-established practice. (237) What is new about these programs is the package, and science lends legitimacy as well as an opportunity for skepticism. Kolata also notes that while "maybe science is telling us that the less-is-more movement is on the right track" (8), individuals — including herself— will continue to practice the "no pain no gain" mantra. She busts various myths like the "fat burning zone" associated with aerobic dance (98–99) and explores a variety of aspects of fitness through this science lens. But she also concludes that she is not one of those "self-appointed people who act like the health police" (261); her "job is just to give you the information that might allow you to think for yourself" (261). In other cases, the weight of science is imbued with authority that is assumed to cross culture and time.

When William J. Broad writes that "this book [*The Science of Yoga*] cuts through the confusion that surrounds modern yoga and describes what science tells us," (5) Broad fails to recognize that this lens of science is hardly free of bias. In fact, he also fails to recognize that his conception of Western science is only one way of considering "science." In *The Yoga Sutras of Patanjali*, Sri Swami Satchidananda describes "the sacred science of Yoga" (vi) that we can "try to practice" (v). Granted, Satchidananda is referring to the Yoga Sutras and the "complete science" presented in these texts by Patanjali Maharishi as he "present[s] the entire Yoga ... a living scripture to illumine our spiritual path" toward liberation (v). However, as much as Broad focuses on Hatha yoga, the physical practice that has been developed in the West over the past several decades, he neglects the influence of yoga spirituality in the teaching and practice of yoga. This science makes its way into unassuming yoga spaces; for instance, *The Yoga Sutras of Patanjali* is required reading and discussion for the level four of YogaFit's training program. Such an element cannot be measured by the science that Broad explores.

Broad recognizes some of the problems with a purely scientific approach in the last few pages of his conclusion. He writes, "what I do know with certainty is that science cannot address, much less answer, many of the most interesting questions in life.... I treasure the scientific method for its insights and discoveries, as well as the wealth of comforts and social advances it has given us. But I question the value of scientism.... Many of yoga's truths go beyond the truths of science" (222). Broadening our perspectives (no pun intended) to include these other modes begins to fill out the bigger picture of yoga, and of fitness, more generally. The fitness picture also fills out when we consider its relationship to sports.

When considering the form and function of "fitness," there is certainly a tension between sports and fitness. Oftentimes, sport is conflated as fitness and fitness is pursued through sports. Kolata's *Ultimate Fitness* leans toward sport with chapters like "Training Lore"; "The Athlete's World"; and "Mount Everest." She "plays" at being an athlete as her love of spinning takes her to new heights. (167) She also notes that many trainers work from the assumption that "anyone who tries, anyone who puts effort into it.... will be trained"(127). But science has shown that not every body can be "trained," not every body will get stronger, leaner, or faster, or even build more endurance. If these are our goals, we might be inclined to give up on exercise and then we might miss out on the other kinds of benefits that exercise has to offer. (130–1)[24]

In many cases, sports might be the avenue through which a woman comes to fitness. Whether through a physical education class where games and sports are often emphasized or through collegiate and professional sport opportunities for women, sports are often where girls and women have the opportunity to discover the power of fitness. This is also where women are taught the dangers of pushing up against the feminized expectations for girls and women. And, obviously, these sporting opportunities are far fewer for women and girls than they are for men and boys. As Wendy Walter-Bailey illustrates in "If These Roads Could Talk: Life as a Woman on the Run," girls and women might be disempowered through sports just much as they are empowered. She writes, "of course, people love to call girls who are in sports 'tomboys' or 'female athletes,' thus negating females the right to own their own fit body" (145). As "tomboys," girls might feel the need to be more "girly" in their lives outside sports, if not in their play. And as "female athletes," there is the constant reminder that girls and women are in a realm of sports that is lower than the "real" realm of sports—where the men play and the girls are not allowed like the Tour de France or the National Football League or where women and men play the same sport but the men dominate and the women are demeaned for their lesser athletic abilities, like in basketball. Instead, women have the Lingerie Football League—a serious sporting competition with serious female athletes packaged as entertainment for men and shown on late-night television.[25]

There are certainly important overlaps between fitness and sports in addition to the marketing overlaps of campaigns like those of Reebok, Pantene, or Cover Girl, for instance. Marketing is a space where women and girls can see their sporting images reflected back to them full of contradictions, stereotypes, and gendered expectations. Describing marketing experts' beliefs (from *USA Today*) Jaana Parviainen argues, "Female tennis players are perfect for product endorsements because their bodies represent an ideal combination of athletic, feminine, youthful, tall and slim." This approach is also supposed to "appeal equally to female and male consumers" (50). So, here, the physical attributes of these particular athletes are the focus, toward selling products. *Women, Sport, and Society* explores some of these important connections between sports and fitness and Roberta J. Park argues that "focusing only on the accomplishments of athletes does not enable one to comprehend the range of what some women have been able to achieve in and through sport and related physical activities" (2). Of course, focusing on the physical attributes, rather than, or in tandem with accomplishments, can be even more problematic.

An empowering consideration of fitness and sport comes from Tara Brabazon's postulations in "Fitness Is a Feminist Issue." She writes, "Aerobics—as a trivialised activity dominated by women—is a case study of how we as feminist theorists can reclaim and rewrite the relationship between sport and politics" (65). Part of her argument hinges on the idea that aerobics is in fact a sport, as illustrated in part by the "arrival of competitive, performance-based aerobics" (67). Thus, just as sports include professional and leisure forms, fitness also includes both "popular and elite participation" (67). If we are looking to define sport outside of "men and balls," the continuum from popular to professional is one important aspect of sport. One of Brabazon's concluding arguments is that "while there are significant questions to ask about what a study of aerobics might add to feminism, there is also a concern with what feminism offers to sports history" (79). As a realm of sport where women are the vast majority of participants, the contributions of aerobics to sport history would be a powerful corrective. Aerobics as sport would also be another opportunity for dominant patriarchal attitudes about sports to further trivialize this activity dominated by women.

Brabazon also considers sport in relation to fitness in terms of the ways in which women's fitness is often equated with disorders. She discusses Marie Campion's definition of anorexia, pointing out that "Campion transforms exercise into a symptom of food-based trauma" (69). As Brabazon points out, if we "exchange the word training for exercise" we can see the contradiction between an understanding of a disease like anorexia and a highly prized social status as athlete. Our assumptions about anorexia are related to problems of mental health while our assumptions about athletes are related, in part, to their mental (and physical) toughness. In order to be a successful athlete or a fit person, Brabazon argues, "a routine must be constructed and continually monitored and updated" (69). This kind of discipline, when exhibited by an athlete, under the care of trainers and other professionals (or not), is evidence of supreme fitness. We celebrate it. But when exercise is seen by Campion as a "'socially acceptable type of purging that receives partial reinforcement from family and friends'" (69), the subject is disempowered rather than lauded as she crosses the finish line. Both must be driven, obsessed. Food is one element where the ironies of form and function challenge an ideal state of fitness.

On the Inescapable Topic of Body Image and Eating Disorders

A junk email: Sender: "SENSA." Subject Line: "Eat Yourself Skinny."

A Love/Social, "Keep It Real Fact" from MissRepresentation.org: "80% of 10-year-old American Girls say they have been on a diet. The number one magic wish for young girls age 11–17 is to be thinner."

"Unfortunately, many people, particularly women, become mired down by the terrible inertia that arises from not liking their own bodies. At its worst, this attitude becomes the diagnosable phenomenon of body dysmorphic disorder. Nia, however, creates the opposite effect — a 'body euphoric' phenomenon."
                    — Debbie and Carlos Rosas, *The Nia Technique* (72)

"I've danced, skated, and boxed my way to understanding that escape from body tyranny is not a matter of revelation but evolution. A crucial factor in this process for me has been the presence and encouragement of other women...." (58)

—Susan Young, "From Ballet to Boxing:
The Evolution of a Female Athlete" (58)

It is easy for me to romanticize and prioritize the positive effects of fitness on myself and others. Perhaps this position is, at least in part, due to the ways in which I constantly struggle to remind myself about the importance of the body beyond image, the priority of the inner before the outer. Research shows that concerns with appearance and the "perfect body" continue to be central to fitness participants as well as instructors and personal trainers (Kennedy and Markula 7–8). None of us who take or teach fitness classes can deny that in addition to feeling good we also want to look good, or at least better than we do without exercise. And there are certainly some who focus on the outer effects of exercise more than the inner, sometimes to the detriment of the inner (and/or outer!). Gina Kolata offers an interesting example which I present more as observation than as critique; she illustrates some of the major problems with ideals of American fitness and its focus on appearance. In the first few pages of her book she admits her obsession with exercise as well as the fact that she uses exercise to keep her weight down. Through her love of spinning she discovers "exhilaration" and through weight training she finds power and the ability to transform her physical appearance. Kolata is honest in her "single transformative moment" (203)—the moment when she notices that her daughter and her high school lacrosse friends are "fast and skilled and incredibly attractive" (204). "This is what weight lifting had done for them, I decided. It had given them strength and exquisite beauty. It's pitiful, I know, to have such thoughts—I'm the mother, for heaven's sake—but I wanted that look, too" (204). The problem is not Kolata's desire for "that look"; this is a desire that isn't about being thin or perfect. But the youth factor of her daughter and friends makes those qualities she observes and desires—firm calves, slim thighs, slender hips, and flat abdomens—more easily achievable. These qualities—firm, flat, slender—are our ideal for "American fitness" for women and girls of all ages. We uphold these patriarchal expectations for ourselves and other women.

The bigger problem with American fitness that this example illuminates is the judgmental attitude that accompanies the ideal of appearance as a marker of fitness. Kolata, who illustrates throughout her book such facts as "some people can gain size but not strength and others can gain strength but not size" (228), also makes a variety of assumptions about fitness based upon the way people look. For instance, after describing the incredible physical prowess of the instructor of her daughter's Spinning training, including a similarity to the teenagers who inspired her to take up lifting, Kolata notes that "the other people in the class did not look nearly so fit" and "only one of them looked truly athletic" (244). These observations come via her daughter, but this does not keep Kolata from critiquing the age, physical appearance, and technical abilities of these newly-certified Johnny G Spinning instructors. Kolata is at least as harsh when it comes to her own appearance; "naturally thin" is not her "fate," which is why she exercises (5). This harsh self-criticism of her own body as not "thin" as well as the presumptive criticism of others' level of fitness based upon appearance illustrate the inescapable topic of body image in the larger discussion of health and fitness.

Body image and eating disorders are strong cultural and psychological forces that are not easy to combat. Our culture (within the U.S. and beyond) won't let go of standards of the physical that determine things like status, power, and desirability. Further, as Tara Brabazon points out, our under-standings of women's fitness are often posed as part and parcel of eating dis-orders. Women, then, are posed as "inferior, weak, sick, and vulnerable" (69). The problems of bodies and disorders are considered to be individual prob-lems, not problems that are connected to larger social and cultural structures. Brabazon recognizes the problems with focusing so much of our understanding of aerobics on its (skewed) relationship with eating disorders; "it becomes lost in an agenda of blaming and shaming for women..." (68). And we, as women, blame and shame ourselves and others, even without realizing that we are doing this.

I cringe when I hear the inspirational, 77-year-old Betty ask her friends if they gained weight over Thanksgiving, or when she lambasts herself for her large dessert the night before. This rail-thin woman who comes to class con-sistently, modifying the movements, and inspiring us all through her com-mitment to fitness and her ability to keep up with those 30 or 50 years younger, is still sometimes focused on her appearance. She wears her uni-form — full on tights, leotard and headband or sometimes a beret — and only sometimes admits she looks good (as she says: for her age). I am frustrated when YMCA members tell me that someone didn't come back to yoga because she heard that it lowers your metabolism (which is true to a certain extent and certainly a contested "fact" of yoga). She wanted to lose weight and sees yoga as counter to such a pursuit. The woman who tells me this has a worried look on her face as she jokes about how her time on the treadmill speeds up her metabolism just to come downstairs and slow it down with yoga. She laughs. I remind her that yoga has many benefits, one of which is balancing out our bodies. She agrees, but there is still an edge of uncertainty, undercut by a desire to stay thin as well as fit.

I am astounded when one of my favorite fitness instructors, and my friend, tells me how she was once hospitalized for anorexia and that she suffered with this disease for most her childhood and adult life and it was finally Nia that saved her life. I am held rapt as Chelsea Roff tells her story in "Starved for Connection: Healing Anorexia Through Yoga." She admits, "If it had not been a roundabout way to burn calories, I never would have walked into that [yoga] class" (79). I am reminded of Jamie who showed me the scars on her knuckles and told me about her struggles with bulimia and anorexia. She also had to have breast reduction surgery; her breast size was intimately connected to her body dysmorphic disorder and her lack of confidence. I am reminded of Mary Kate and Erin and Trish who obsessed about the number of workouts and the calories burned, who taught multiple classes and then went for a jog, the weight room, a swim. I am reminded of the stories of big-city instructors snorting coke before class to keep up their energy. I am reminded of the half-joking observations some of us make about how we workout so we can eat. And there is satisfaction in the food that follows a good workout.

Whenever I hear anyone negatively refer to their body, I am on the instant defensive. I am reminded of the ways in which I judge my physical imperfections harshly. The way my mother's self-criticisms scratch at the edges of my brain as she thinks she might finally be happy if she could just lose 10 more pounds, those last five pounds, that fat under her arms, that roll around her middle. She wishes she could look like the stars—those she knows have plastic surgery and personal chefs and every beauty product produced by man. I tell her that she cannot judge herself against those images, that she cannot obsess about those parts of her body that she sees as a problem. She knows. I try to remind myself not to do this either. I try not to look in the mirror and judge how fat this or that part looks—the way the fat bulges from my sports bra, the rub of my inner thighs, that same roll around the middle. I try to let fitness sedate my compulsive overeating. It creeps at the edges.

In a culture and society based upon—obsessed with—image, it is impossible to escape the many ways in which we love to hate our bodies. The well-worn example of Tina Fey's spoof of this phenomenon—as the "mean girls" comically evaluate their physical shortcomings, criticizing the minute details of their calves, skin, shoulders—illustrates the petty obsessiveness that body image can evoke.[26] They are parts, not whole. But this example also reminds us of its salience since we can all laugh at the joke even as we cannot escape the way it plays out in our lives. I am reminded that many women won't step foot in a gym or a fitness center, or any kind of fitness space, because "that's for skinny girls." I am reminded of those who feel fat and lumpy and hide in the back of the classroom. Some women resist exposing themselves to a space that they perceive as hostile. Bodies are barriers to seeking fitness. With consistency, some are transformed into stronger, leaner versions of themselves. Some bodies resist physical/visually recognizable transformation and some of these bodies still experience transformations of life and mind.

As we search for fitness—a healthy, non-distorted view of our own bodies—we are also inundated by images of bodies that are only achievable through eating disorders juxtaposed against the reality of overweight and obese American bodies that are also achieved through eating disorders. This fact is well-recognized but not so easily rectified. It is another irony that poor body image and eating disorders should plague the fitness of a population with plenty. And these disorders disrupt fitness—offering false ideas of fitness—ideas that fitness is all about image and not about the way we feel and function. Body image and eating disorders are fitness plagues—mind/body disruptions—cured by a shift in consciousness. This book explores the signs and symptoms of what Brabazon describes as "disordered eating" as well as its antidotes.

The Language of Fitness

"The hyperconsciousness of our bodies in the contained studio gives language a different spin. The teacher's instructions begin to sound like a chant, and as we move into the class, most of what she expresses is communicated nonverbally. Language leaks away, leaving us with an unfamiliar, momentary clarity."
—Victoria Boynton, "Women's Yoga" (120)

I have never felt that I had much talent or ability for learning languages, but the language of fitness has come easily to me. It makes sense. It is stable but also always changing. It varies from format to format and place to place but everyone who does step speaks a similar language and everyone who teaches Group Active speaks the same language. The weight room has its own language. And everyone who teaches Nia speaks the same language. And everyone who does yoga speaks a variation on a language that combines English translations and instructions with ancient Sanskrit. Everyone who has taken a fitness class understands the basic language and expectations even if this language feels foreign at first and even if the movements feel awkward and the space feels uncomfortable. Learning the language(s) of fitness is a starting point. The language of fitness manifests itself in choreography. To write choreography and to read choreography one must be versed in the language of fitness. And even then, one is not guaranteed to be able to read someone else's written version, especially without a key. These are building blocks — permission for conscious, creative re-construction.

The language of fitness is complicated — it is simultaneously mathematical, descriptive, kinesthetic, verbal, visual, and musical. It requires an ear and eye and muscle memory for layers. It can be learned in part and in whole. It can be used and it can be transformed. It is a tool of communication and it is a tool for expression. It is a building block for movement and a method of organization. When non-verbal, the body speaks, points directions, indicates depth, reach. When written, it can vary greatly according to the way the writer expresses this complicated language and it may not make sense without first understanding the formula, terminology, and abbreviations. It takes unlocking and it takes reconstruction. To record the entire experience of choreography on a flat page is to record the essence, the foundation. The reader/instructor brings it to life through movement.

Some moves are mimetic like imitating a lawnmower pull or doing "scissors." Some are metaphor, making comparisons like: now you are a lion. Some are synecdoche, where part represents the whole; we tell participants to put on their high heel shoes to imagine the foot position of a Latin dancer. And some are metonymy like when "Africa" stands in to describe a hip movement derived from an African dance move; we refer to a continent to tell participants to push their hip back and alternating arm forward. There is a basic fitness language derived from the foundations of dance and step aerobics (which was, of course, originally developed from dance and other forms of movement). Names for movements are often functional, literal. Knee lift. Step touch. Movements also take the names of their shapes or associations. Step moves might be simple descriptions like "basic step" or "V step" or they might become stylized like "the matador" or "the cowboy." Dance moves are names drawn from classic staples to descriptive images. Chassé to snake arms to the Running Man. They have the least uniformity and are the most difficult to cue. But we get used to the names as much as the movement. Sway. Tap. Shake. Breathe. The common language is only one aspect of instruction and it combines instruction and art. And it is also a science.

In the language of fitness one number holds infinite significance. All counts are bundled in 8s. The constant of the number 8 — my favorite number for its infinite loop, its roundness, the linking of two circles or the flowing of one movement — provides a stability for the mathematical variations. Two counts of four. Four counts of two. Eight counts times four equals a phrase. Thirty-two counts. Everything is even, everything repeats in predictable and map-able patterns. When we count moves we rarely count higher than 8. And, as common standard, we count down so we all know how many repe-

titions or steps are left. Mixer music produces predictable 32-counts for
instructors to use and companies like The Step Company (BTS) and Zumba
manufacture music specific to its programs, molded to its movements and
purposes.

Certain fitness programs might use and adapt language in ways particular
to their program. For instance, the July 2012 release for Group Groove includes
the term "Groove-tacular" in their marketing and promotion. Zumba has
begun the trend of silent cueing, a quality that makes it easy to transfer this
program from one country to another, from one language location to the
next. Talented instructors master the use of the non-verbal cue while talented
performers model the way Zumba is "supposed" to look. Participants are
expected to follow along until they know enough to begin to execute the
movements correctly. This is a language that is largely lost in translation, a
language that becomes internalized, and a language that might not even be
used for demonstration or instruction. This silence is not the same as that
which Boynton describes in the yoga studio. Both are shared understandings
of expectations but with yoga there is a hyperconsciousness that may never
be met, while Zumba breeds an unconsciousness that might be transcended.
In many fitness programs there is repetition without thoughtfulness, movement without feeling. But at least words can remind participants how to do
what they are doing and how to do it safely. Words can remind us that we
should be feeling, not simply doing, and that there is a purpose beyond burning calories. But our words might also reinforce the calorie-burning goals.
Perhaps there is more of an opportunity for a mind/body connection in the
silent cueing of Zumba.[27] At the very least the body is speaking different variations of silence.

Translation is most interesting and problematic in yoga. In my early yoga
training I essentially ignored Sanskrit terms. I figured I wouldn't remember
them anyway and thought I would alienate my fitness participants. When I
take a yoga class with an instructor who incorporates Sanskrit, I most often
feel annoyed at her pretentious approach. While it is an important reminder
of yoga's ancient roots, coming from an American yogi wearing the latest
overpriced yoga clothing, it feels more like a practice in Orientalism than it
does a practice of cultural connection and understanding. It is often an attempt
at authenticity that feels shallow and can make students feel uncomfortable.
But as I began to learn more, a deeper understanding developed of why the
language of yoga might be important to know and useful to include in class.
Some poses have been named in English in ways that obscure their connections
to other poses. There is a simplicity and beauty to Sanskrit and it is a connection across borders. But I have yet to move past two or three words.

Trikonasana and *tadasana* are about the limit to my Sanskrit, and I remember those not only because of their simplicity but because the triangle is my favorite yoga pose and the mountain is my favorite yoga symbol.

Language can be welcoming or off-putting, helpful instruction or mindless chatter. It can complement a fitness routine or clutter the space. It can make connections.

Fitness Spaces

> People "have sought and are finding meaning and community in diverse sites of physical movement and fitness: gyms, dance studios, skating rinks, boxing rings, and more."
> — Jo Malin, *My Life at the Gym* (14)

> "The studio is a respite from busy-ness, a constructed space apart from the business of thinking, doing, having. It is an undoing place, a place beyond the words, sentences, and automatic thinking that governs our ordinary experience."
> — Victoria Boynton, "Women's Yoga" (120)

> "Women who occupied the city streets and rural roads to win their right to vote did so with a sense of ownership and entitlement. They were not temporarily passing through the public sphere but were *in it* in order to be *of it*."
> — Jaime Schultz, "The Physical Is Political" (31; original emphasis).

In Body Pump or Group Power we claim our space, stack our equipment. In Zumba we squeeze in. In yoga we relax and clear our minds; our mat is our four-cornered world. In Nia we "step in" and embrace the opportunity for movement. We find our spot. Sometimes that spot moves. Sometimes we are forced to move. We can choose but we can rarely control the spaces where fitness happens. We have created these spaces or these spaces have been prefabricated, remodeled, borrowed, or constructed. Fitness space is a luxury. Even so, rooms are often too hot, too cold, too small, too large, too many mirrors, not enough mirrors. Inevitably, a room will be freezing cold for yoga and then burning hot for cardio. The floor will be too dirty for bare feet or slippery from humidity or the drips of sweat from the previous class. We wipe the floor, put on extra layers of clothing, drink extra water, prop the door open, squeeze extra close. We make fitness happen where we are. We have to make space in our schedules for fitness to happen and we have to make space in our heads to remember the importance of fitness in our (busy) lives.

One of the beauties of fitness is that it can happen anywhere, that it does not have to be contained by predetermined spaces. Certainly some kinds of spaces are better for some kinds of fitness and some kinds of fitness need certain kinds of spaces. But fitness can be done in a windowless basement or a penthouse with sky lights, an elementary school gym or an empty lot. And yet, there is something to be said for a beautiful, inspiring space. A physical environment can affect the mental processes and physical body positively, negatively, or neutrally. Attention to lights, arrangement, size, mirrors, colors, equipment placement, instructor visibility, and other factors may all influence a fitness experience.

Experiencing fitness in and through nature is inspiring, calming, rejuvenating. And yet, as Jacquelyn Allen-Collinson notes:

> Exercising outdoors — whether rural or urban — as opposed to indoors, does engender lived-body vulnerabilities. At times rural isolation seems to hold more danger: distance from people, safety and sources or help, challenging terrain, encounters with animals. But then the urban harbors a set of specific dangers, especially at night: dark alleys and underpasses, doorways where men can lurk and lunge out, drunks, stalkers, gangs of men and youths.

Because of violent realities and cultural construction, these may be fears of women in these spaces regardless of whether they are working out, working, or just going from point A to point B. As dangerous as outside spaces can be, they can also be empowering, even intrinsic to one's experience of fitness and life. As Allen-Collinson continues:

> But being outdoors is an intrinsic part of running for me (indoor treadmill running is a dire last resort): facing all the elements in the fresh air, battling against vicious wind, stinging hail and pelting rain, sinking in fresh snow, glistening in high summer sun, melting into dark night, coursing over fields eerie in silvery moonlight, running alongside the heavy beat of flying swans [290].

These qualities are lived, bodily experience, merging observation and movement. These are qualities experienced through fitness and through the kinds of recreation experiences that fitness can help prepare us for — hiking, backpacking, canoeing, mountain biking. There is potential for danger and for enjoyment and empowerment.

Spaces can also be intimidating or empowering indoors. Weight rooms, for instance, are notorious for their lack of female-friendly attributes, including the male gaze. Women often feel uncomfortable, alone. Even the judgment of the female gaze can be intimidating, especially in spaces where gossip and unhealthy or unattainable ideas of fitness reign. As argued in "Large Women's Experiences of Exercise," "Segregated to a separate training space, the large women [in this research study] already experienced that their bodies were problematic and wrong as judged by others" (123). They have already been ostracized; then, special programs create private spaces, reinforcing that ostracism. While segregated spaces are often assumed to be automatically empowering — like the women-only spaces of Curves or other women's gyms — these spaces can also be oppressive. As Louise Mansfield argues in "Fit, Fat and Feminine? The Stigmatization of Fat Women in Fitness Gyms," gyms are "commonly thought of as an intimidating place for those who were not well versed in the fitness regimes and those who did not look good/fit" (86). Certain spaces, like gyms, might assume a certain level of knowledge in order to be comfortable, let alone even enter such spaces in the first place. Walking into a weight room without knowledge of equipment, let alone one's own body, is intimidating, overwhelming, sometimes impossible. Walking into a studio full of women you don't know is sometimes even more difficult. Men may be just as intimidated walking into group fitness spaces as women are walking into the weight room; these are gendered spaces. But men are conditioned to own spaces as if they belong everywhere while women are taught to fade to the edges.

Increasingly, fitness spaces, are online, virtual, or digital. They are found on social networks like Facebook and in Blog and Twitter and Pinterest form. Many such fitness spaces are explored throughout this book; many like Decolonizing Yoga and Fit Femininity challenge traditional ideas about fitness. But many online spaces also reinforce ideas about fitness that keep us boxed into ideas and ideals about certain kinds of bodies. For instance, measuring ourselves (our weight, body fat percentage, bicep circumference) as well as our intake of food and output of calories is a helpful way for some individuals to approach literally or figuratively getting in shape. But these tools also keep us focused on the numbers and distracted from the less tangible benefits of fitness. For instance, Myfitnesspal.com and the Super Tracker at usda.gov ("My foods. My fitness. My health.") will help you keep track of your caloric intake and expenditure. You can count and account. And many health and fitness resources can be found in this space, whether one elects to become a member or not.

Fitness is ultimately about owning access and practicing flexibility. If your fitness has to happen in a small, confined space, it does. If it has to happen on a wide-open grass lawn, it can. If it happens with chairs, it works. If not everyone is following, it can still work. If you don't have all the right equipment, you can make do. Fitness fits as long as we make room for it. Clear some literal and/or physical space. *How much space do you really need?* Some of us make the physical environment through imagination. The physical space does not matter so much because we've made figurative space in our heads. We breathe in the choreography. We imbibe the music. We relish the silence. We find what we need and let go of that which cannot be controlled. Maybe we complain. But we are drawn back to fitness spaces as we continue to find ourselves.

Ultimately we need only our own bodies to work our bodies. Insanity practices this principle to the extreme, but belly dancing practices it as principle. Al-Fawi explains: "Little space is needed for belly dancing, for its true space is the body itself. The movements of belly dancing are intense and meditation-like, the dancer seeming to be illuminating her inner space rather than needing space outside her" (59). Meditative movement, whether for socialization, performance, or exercise can be a powerful tool toward fitness and transformation.

Perhaps the most important space associated with fitness is the space that we open in our heads and our lives and our hearts through fitness. When we let go, we make room for new experiences. When we clear some space, we have more space to move. More space to live, more space to breathe. More space to work.

Two

Tools and Trade

The Work of Fitness

"For us — like so many others who struggled to be fit — movement had become work. It was donkey kicks. Sit-ups. Push-ups. Repetition. Drudgery. We were like wild horses, captured and domesticated, that pulled a plow."
— Debbie Rosas and Carlos Rosas, *The Nia Technique* (15)

"Within the restrictions of the post–Fordist, temporarily employed workforce, a controlled body is both a metonymy and mask for a controlled life."
— Tara Brabazon, "Fitness Is a Feminist Issue" (70)

Most of the people I know who teach fitness do it because they love it. Some make a good living. Some do it for the gym membership. Some support their families. Many of us teach to stay active and connected. Some have a supplemental income. And fitness has its own set of celebrity personalities — fitness stars. Their work is a mix of fitness and entertainment. There's money to be made and fame to take advantage of. But regardless of why we teach, teaching fitness is work. It is work as employment, as a "workout," as a mental and physical effort. It is a service and requires clients/participants and some kind of infrastructure. As part of a business, or a community, the work of fitness is more than a work/out.

As a form of work, fitness is certainly not without its ironies. The idea of "working out" is a luxury in a culture where many of us are increasingly sedentary, obese. We sit, we drive, we take elevators and escalators, and then we get on the treadmill for our workout. If our work were physical would we need this workout? Maybe. As Brabazon argues, "Exercise and fitness, from the 1980s through to the present, has been medication for the physical changes resulting from technology, such as cars, elevators, computers and the other accoutrements of post-industrialisation" (66). Exercise and fitness are a sign of the times. The physical exertion of work can be complicated, complemented, and substituted through fitness. As William J. Broad notes in *The Science of Yoga*, we became interested in fitness when we shifted to an urban, sedentary lifestyle. At the same time, we see the growth of the fitness industry that is, according to Debbie Rosas and Carlos Rosas, shaping us into physical beings akin to domesticated animals. And if this is the state of America, then the work of fitness professionals is one of utmost importance. Because "fitness" is an ideology, a way of living and being, a state of mind as much as it is a state of body, there is much at stake in this work. And the state of the work that we do in fitness can impact our state of fitness.

The employment-related work of fitness takes constant innovation, trainings, certifications. It requires equipment, sustenance, and planning. Teaching fitness takes time and money and the working conditions vary greatly in the world of fitness. Even in my limited experience my pay has differed drastically depending upon where I am working. I typically make $10 to $13 per hour — the hour I am teaching class — and I am typically not paid, or compensated in any way, for the time that it takes to plan and practice my routines, interact with participants before and after class, attend trainings, or engage in self-education about my practice. There are some exceptions. For instance, some of the facilities where I have taught have paid an extra 10 minutes or so before and after class and some have paid at least part of mandatory, encouraged, or optional training fees. Most facilities provide a free membership to the instructor; some provide benefits for family or partner memberships. In some cases, family benefits are being decreased. For instance, at a private club in Oregon (in 2001) I had a family membership, but when I started working at the YMCA (in 2009) in Maine the family benefits were being cut. Since many fitness instructors teach only a class or two or teach a lot of classes and rely upon their benefits to provide childcare or swimming lessons for their children or rely upon the scant income to make ends meet, such a change typically impacts an instructor's income more than it impacts the profits of the facility. If an instructor needs childcare while she teaches, her margin of profit is even lower. She may be just breaking even.

In fitness work, efficiency and skill can increase money earned by decreasing effort exerted. As a fitness instructor gains experience, she needs to put less time into creating routines and much less time (if any) is devoted to practicing new material. But this can also cause complacency, a dangerous trait in fitness instruction when we rely upon old habits rather than renewed knowledge. And acceptable standards change. What used to be safe and effective when Jane Fonda's videos hit the market is quite different from the tested and reviewed products that Body Training Systems produces, for instance. However, with solid skills and a conscious approach, instructors can teach safely and effectively without the need for constant innovation, mandatory training requirements, or new accessories.

The rise of manufactured fitness means that fitness instructors might have to put in more (or less!) work — memorizing routines. This work varies from instructor to instructor; we memorize in different ways. And far more *work* goes into a manufactured fitness program than an experienced fitness instructor's own choreography. Development, testing, safety check, taping, design, packaging, marketing — all before it is viewed, memorized, practiced, and delivered. And all of this inspires the work of the workout. While manufactured fitness is more structured, the call for innovation — for something new with each new release — is even more urgent. These programs have also changed working power dynamics within the industry. As Jaana Parviainen argues, this kind of franchising principle "has generated a new kind of hierarchy in the fitness culture between female instructors and female license owners" (56). The power of the fitness supervisor (one who manages programs and personnel at a facility) — who now answers to the brand as well as the facility (and maybe a board of trustees or other power structures) — has decreased and, as a result, an instructor's power has decreased as well. She has to pay more to do her work and perhaps she has more work to do; and perhaps she has less control over how she does her work. She is a part of the larger structure.

Tara Brabazon illuminates this larger structure when she argues that "what is considered a popular sport or leisure in a particular period shadows the understanding of work. How women are incorporated into physical culture is an indicator of their place and role in the contemporary workplace and citizenship" (66). In other words, women, who are marginalized in the political economy — they make less and work more — are also marginalized in terms of their fitness choices — the sports and leisure that they engage in (or don't engage in). They have less access, fewer opportunities, and less time for fitness; they also have to navigate stereotypes about laziness and dependence which do not fit with "fitness." Further, women who do not fit into idealized images of fitness (lean, sculpted, light) stand out as examples of women who are devalued because they have, as many critics note, "let themselves go." The word choice reveals the judgment. Where control of one's self is highly valued, the body becomes the evidence of such control. A lack of a workout seems to mirror the idea that there is a lack of a work ethic and this assumption is clouded by a lack of an understanding of oppression and privilege.[1]

But the problem is bigger than just the inequalities that women find in the economy more generally. As Brabazon explains: "the political environment in which we live, with a rollback in welfare, health privatisation [sic], and reduction in full-time, stable employment, means that we are all 'passing,' thinking that attention to body management will replace the need for collective political struggles by women against neo-conservative governments" (75). These economic conditions most impact those at the margins of our society — the poor and working classes, immigrants, the disabled — those whose work bolsters the fitness and "collective political struggles" and pursuits of the middle and upper classes. Brabazon explains that the white middle class is able to "'consume' fitness as a part of their lifestyle, [while] the working class is socially and spatially excluded from infrastructure and facilities, including those promoting health." Most importantly, she argues that "health problems are created not by bad choices from individuals but by *structural poverty* and *inequality*...." (70; my emphasis). Thus, part of the work of fitness is to change these structural inequalities. In this section, I consider some of the ways in which we might do such fitness work — in and out of academia — toward awareness, education, and social justice.

Sketches: Instructors

"Group exercise instructors are integral in creating an atmosphere in which all of their participants — regardless of their reason for being in the class — can enjoy and succeed."
"Instructors are pivotal in the process of creating an emotionally and physically healthy environment that has the potential to empower."
— Kristine Newhall, "'You Spin Me Right Round, Baby'" (72)

Fitness instructors are an interesting group. For most of my early life I saw them as a stereotyped group, as a group of flighty, bubbly women or pumped-up, vapid men, even if my limited experience did not fit the image in my head. Later, when teaching college composition classes I would use the "fitness instructor" to discuss stereotypes as well as writing approaches. But I found that, for the most part, people didn't really hold stereotypes of fitness instructors simply because they had not thought that much about this group. I have spent much time with fitness instructors and not only are they a diverse group, they are often also highly committed, motivated women who work more than one job and have a mountain of responsibilities. Some work harder. Some are divas. Some are wounded. Some teach as a hobby, others as a living. Some are certainly less committed or less mentally or creatively gifted. Some are stay-at-home moms with the need for outside work and adult contact. Some approach their teaching with love, others with rote obligation. Like any group, fitness instructors are deeper than an image.[2]

More than once I have been told that I don't look like a fitness instructor. Most of the time this is meant as a compliment and I try not to over-think it. After all, this has been an element of pride. This is one of the reasons I wanted to be a fitness instructor in the first place, one of the reasons I persist. I have wanted to model a different picture of fitness. It doesn't really bother me when a participant approaches me after class and hopes I won't be offended when she asks me if I have heard of "wheat belly." As she explains the idea, I am reminded of some of the stuff I read about wheat online and then I realize that she is referring to the weight I have recently gained, which has settled around my middle. The instructor's body is always on display. A few months later, as I lose the 10 to 15 pounds that I had gained, the compliments come easily from my participants. My body represents their own insecurities and triumphs. Sometimes I am their mirror.

My fellow fitness instructors are overwhelmingly (white) women, in popular culture and in my geographic locales (even as men dominate prominent "trainer" roles). In thirteen years of teaching at fitness centers, gyms, university recreation centers, community centers, the YMCA, and private studios, I have known only a handful of male instructors and just as few instructors who are women of color. Until recently, the male instructors I knew only taught abs classes or bootcamp-style classes. The men mostly worked the weight room. They were the personal trainers and very few would take group fitness classes, fewer would teach them. But men who do teach fitness classes are inevitably popular. Many are very good at what they do, but many are also emblematic of the power of male authority, even in, or especially in, predominantly female spaces. Many women will more readily submit to the will of a male instructor (even when flamboyantly gay) without realizing that they are more accepting of male authority. And, often, men are a special commodity. For instance, I got an invitation to participate in a Zumbathon and in the e-mail there was a particular call for male instructors, in order to "honor" Beto, the founder, guru, and God of Zumba. A follow-up e-mail said that they were still searching voraciously for a male instructor. Such desperate attempts to involve — and sometimes elevate — men in activities that are dominated by women devalue the women. But most women (and men) just want a good workout and gender is not so important. A good, solid instructor is what we desire. And some men are brave enough to frequent the group fitness arena.

Most of my friends over the years have come from a population of fitness instructors, whether this friendship is strictly confined to the realm of fitness or whether it develops outside of the gym. We develop bonds with each other through our common interests, through our common population. Some of us are territorial, some insecure. Some of us work really hard to be our best and others of us think we don't need much practice. Some of us — many of us — are amazing. Despite the common moves, music, language, training, each of us develops our own style and has our own strengths and weaknesses. And with a few exceptions, I have found that fitness instructors share with each other, support each other, and motivate each other.

The instructors I've trained, my shadows — those who survive more than a few steps in the training process — are solid. Alyssa, Eleni, Ashley, Shauna, Sakura. They make me so proud but it is ultimately their work that makes them excellent instructors. They sometimes internalize a phrase I overuse; they use similar methods and combinations. They have their own favorite moves and variations. They are recognizable as my trainees. They are methodical, balanced. They love a challenge and seek perfection.

Alyssa takes on "tapless" step and amazes me as she seamlessly moves through her routine. She gets inspired by "Step Junkie" and creates her own videos. She is awesome. She takes on Turbo Kick and other fitness programs. She goes to school full-time — science or engineering or something like that. And she is a fantastic seamstress. She gets married. She bakes and cooks and posts her recipes. She grows. She starts working a real, full-time job and stops teaching fitness classes. She'll be back.

Within a few months, Sakura learned step and kickboxing. It came easily to her. She worked hard to be perfect. She took on yoga. I was struck when I noticed that she was translating all the yoga pose names back and forth from Japanese to English. What I assumed was easy for her was more than hard work and dedication. It was bridging cultural gaps. It was struggling for self.

Erin searches for ways to amp up her routine. She makes more challenging combinations and increases the beats per minute. She practices perfection. She accepts nothing less. I wonder if it lasts. If the music is too fast, the movements are incomplete, hasty.

Pam is forty-something, has five kids, looks incredible. She makes Zumba moves looks easy. She cues very little and sometimes is just off the beat. But people flock to her classes. She's passionate about Zumba, takes many trainings, and enjoys the time she spends teaching.

Only Stephanie can pull off the skort. Her long legs were apparently made for such a silly clothing style. And even with two risers she often seems too tall for her step. But she finds her rhythm and we follow her fun, interesting, challenging choreography. Hers was the only class I really liked at my old YMCA. She was the only instructor whose class I really liked to take. In most cases I just prefer my own classes. Stephanie and I were on the same page.

Ashley makes no mistakes. She is solid. She researches cures for cancer by day. Her commitment to fitness is readily apparent. She is gorgeous and grounded. She takes her teaching seriously.

Kari's warmth is welcoming. She is earthly and ephemeral. She creates a space that welcomes us but does not intrude on our transition from life into the studio. She moves like Danielle, my favorite Nia instructor. She is genuine, relaxed, and a bit detached (or at least it's tough for me to break through). She believes and practices what she teaches. I feel invisible in her presence, disappearing behind my eyes and in front of hers.

Joanne is one of those people who doesn't have much rhythm and can't find the beat. Without these skills it is pretty difficult to be a group fitness instructor. But, as a department supervisor, she did all of the trainings. She worked to learn the skills even though they did not come naturally. And she found her niche. She found that yoga and cycling were forms she enjoyed and forms she enjoyed teaching. Neither required a beat. She has excelled.

Trish is hard core. Too much for me, but I have much respect for her. I don't know how she gets so low, how she does so many reps. I don't know why she feels the need to show off. She yells and has a big personality. She dresses like a diva and acts her role. She, too, loves choreography and has a storehouse of it in her head. She studied history in college but she chose the fitness route. But she sacrifices safety for something I can't quite understand. She is on stage. And yet she loves what she does and she genuinely wants to help people get/stay fit. She is a force.

Danielle embodies love, passion, and compassion. She is joy in motion. She is present and reaches out to everyone in the room. Nia is not the same without her. As I take Nia classes from other instructors, I wonder if it is Nia I love or if this feeling is actually just love for Danielle. She teaches me so much; she transforms me. She transforms us.

Tammy is bubbly and bouncy and silly and smiling. She does it all. She reminds us that she is 50 because if she didn't remind us, we would forget. She sometimes spaces her choreography — she does teach a handful of different classes every week — but she laughs it off and we laugh with her. She motivates and inspires without being fake. Her smile is genuine and, as director, she listens to members' complaints thoughtfully. She also models how to handle limitations and set boundaries. She supports her instructors in and out of the studio.

Becky is beautiful — stereotypically and in actuality. Tall, blond, shapely; she has it all. She glistens, covered in sweat, still smiling, eyes sparkling. We takes her classes, in part, to watch her move. She opens her arms and her reach goes wall to wall. But she is down to earth and she works hard. She memorizes BTS programming quickly and as a tester she can sell anything.

She makes it fun. She is phenomenal at cueing — one of the best I've ever known so it is always a pleasure to take her class. She is always on time and gives verbal and visual indicators. She takes her moves big — from one side of the room to the other — and makes everyone feel comfortable.

Beth fills the room with her enthusiasm and humor. Her skills, or at least her reservoir of moves is limited. She dusts off the same old combos over and over again. But we barely notice. She has us laughing, breathing heavily. She has us kicking and punching and moving and we hardly notice when the hour is up.

Heidi's eyes shine when she teaches. She sparkles from within and I have to resist the urge to be completely overwhelmed by her inner/outer beauty. I am disenchanted when, one night, I can see the strain; I can see through the attempts to appear energetic and unfettered. And I can relate; I too am over-scheduled and over-committed. There is something that lurks beneath pushing her to embellish a jump or exaggerate a subtle movement. And yet she brings joy to her work. She motivates. She moves effortlessly, making it look easy. Each class I am more charmed.

Val flows from one move to the next effortlessly and only sometimes awkwardly. She commands our attention and encourages us. We do crazy things in her classes like dragging ourselves across the floor. She pushes us. She does her own thing, always taking new trainings, always adapting the new to her style, practiced through more than 30 years of teaching fitness classes.

Jane checks her form — or is it her hair — through furtive side-glances. She loves squats. She mixes them with goofy, playful flourishes. She is reliable, versatile, energetic.

* * *

I am serious. I have fun, but I also have a plan. I can deviate from the plan when needed, and there is always some need for deviation — time, temperature, ability. Innovation — as I plan or execute my choreography — is a must. Sometimes I plan carefully, especially for more complicated step or dance choreography. But, for years I have walked into class with little more than a general plan. Yoga and kickboxing just flow into a balanced class, almost effortlessly. But it is an effort to be fresh and enthusiastic. It helps to team teach. It helps to remember the love.

I love the predictability and endless variation in step, the way that all of the pieces fit into place seamlessly. With the right transitions and complementary combinations of moves, class is a puzzle that we unravel together.

Creating a step routine is like assembling that puzzle — making room for surprises, for moments. Teaching step is an art of precision and requires impeccable cueing but it is also a challenge to make a puzzle out of a box.

I love the variation and room for creativity in kickboxing; I embrace the power that flows through punches and kicks even if it is only an imitation of the fight. I love weaving together a routine that travels in all directions, combines styles and movements, and engages the entire body. My yoga students laugh at the transition from "Zen Sarah" to Kick-ass Sarah"; it happens in the 10 minutes between classes.

I love the rules that govern Pilates and yoga, the sets of poses and postures that need to be organized and assembled toward a set of goals. I aim for flow. Mat Pilates must be consistent and precise. Yoga Fit's "mountains" and "valleys" create a vision of class that makes sense to me and has as much flexibility as it does structure. The pieces fit together and match breath. Both feel like a science in ways that other fitness classes don't. Both work mind and body.

I love my classes the most but I also enjoy taking classes, always learning from other instructors. I love witnessing their art. Counting along and cueing myself without thinking, I inadvertently memorize the steps and notice the small errors that other participants don't usually notice. I appreciate perfection. And, yet, I never see a mistake as a weakness; we all make mistakes. Perfection is nearly impossible. But it is satisfactory, sometimes magical.

Dance is more magical. I love teaching belly dancing, watching women drop their inhibitions at the door, or during the warm-up, or finally as we relax onto our mats at the end of class. I love crafting songs and routines, choreographing movements and music and finding ways to translate movement into fitness. Certain songs move me and I can't get them out of my head until I start to make them move. And Group Groove embeds itself in my brain and body, aching to move. There is freedom and structure and a connection between mind and body. There is pleasure in endless variation.

I love stepping into class without a plan, with only a vague idea of what storehouse I will pull from. I love stepping into class with a crafted routine. I love teaching and I can't help but put this love into every class. I can only hope that it is the love that participants take with them and bring back the next time.

Building a Toolbox: Interdisciplinary Praxis

In the world I inhabit for most of my work, using ideas from other people's work requires citation. Plagiarism is the evil word reserved for those who steal other people's ideas — intentionally or unintentionally — without citation.

And while we are expected to collaborate and build upon other people's ideas, we are also expected to critique. Originality is mandatory. Most adhere to a strictly disciplinary set of tools. I approach this work with a variety of tools between and among disciplines and aim to reveal patterns and inspire ideas and activism. This methodology is a lot like Hip Hop's technique of sampling. It is a borrowing (and perhaps manipulation) of any theory, method, example, or idea that fits a particular need — in the theory, the argument, the process, the classroom. Sampling provides context for community and culture while it might also be oppositional on a structural level. Academic conventions require citation but sampling speaks to the reality of interdisciplinary methodology — some sources demand their due; others need only be recognized as familiar in a shared, collective culture.[3]

In fitness, we are taught to pull from a variety of sources for our teaching. We are encouraged to "steal" a move or combo we particularly like — to teach it as is or to innovate upon it and make it our own. We learn, adapt, incorporate. The more fitness training and knowledge one has (and with the skills to put that knowledge to use), the more an experienced instructor can teach spontaneously and plan meticulously, from the many pieces and scripts in our heads and the many movements embedded in our muscles. As a new teacher, we have less of a storehouse to pull from. We slowly learn from observation and repetition. We create combos, we put them together into routines. We practice those combos and routines over and over again. It becomes second nature; we repeat and innovate, over and over. Sometimes these can get stale, but our continuing education — formal and informal — will refresh our toolbox periodically.

While this approach to instruction has largely changed due to the dominance and predominance of manufactured fitness forms (we are discouraged from misusing patented fitness programming), even if we do not create our choreography, we need a toolbox of practical knowledge and skills as well as the ability to cue correctly and the ability to memorize choreography and to read the language in which it is written. Teacher-training programs that teach a set of skills to teach a formula of fitness classes might not always be teaching versatility or creativity, but they are still teaching a set of tools and creating a kind of toolbox that could be applied outside of the sometimes-constricting choreography or formula. For instance, programs like Zumba or Body Training Systems (BTS), teach instructors (or potential instructors) only how to teach their particular program(s), but skills of delivery can be adaptable across forms. What I learn in one training will apply in other fitness settings. Other trainings provide other kinds of knowledge. Nia teaches about more than just the learning of a toolbox and the teaching of a particular program; it seeks to transform one's relationship to fitness. YogaFit also has transformative effects on teachers/trainers. Every training I attend begins and ends with stories of transformation, of continuing works in progress; we come back for further training because of these transformative impacts. We keep working it out.

* * *

There are also a variety of tools that we can use as instructors. Like music, choreography, and cueing. Choreography is dependent upon music, as well as a variety of other factors including what kind of class it is, who the participants are, what the space is, what equipment is needed or available. Regardless of these constraints, choreography is a mixture of the structures of the craft and the instructor's base of knowledge and experience. In most of what I teach I create my own choreography — before class when doing song-specific choreography and during class when I teach to mixer music. How I cue these movements is another tool as I can inspire and instruct. Together music, choreography, and cuing create the movement and experience of the class; freedom over these elements can give an instructor much control over her class.

The creativity involved in choosing the music for a fitness class is impeded by a growing market for fitness music and a growing role of manufactured fitness in the music business. But there may be a new opportunity as well. As a 2013 *Wall Street Journal* article argues: "The New Music Gurus" are "Group Fitness Instructors" and the "New DJs" are "Fitness Gurus." The author, Katherine Rosman, argues that with the "waning impact of traditional radio on the music-buying public ... fitness companies are increasingly getting into the music business." In part, this means that record companies have a new source of revenue as others wane. Rosman poses this as a reciprocal relationship: the music companies are "cutting deals with fitness chains" and "exercise businesses are trying to cut licensing deals with music companies in order to package and sell workout songs in much the same way that film and television executives do with sound tracks." All of this is happening on the level of manufactured fitness and Zumba is in the forefront as it depends upon its numbers to increase its music business power ("14 million people take at least one Zumba class per week globally," notes Rosman). Zumba's co-founder and chief executive, Alberto Perlman, describes Zumba as both a fitness company and a music company and has partnered with Universal Music Group to produce an album "Zumba Fitness Dance Party" (Rosman). Rosman also credits Zumba with reviving the career of rapper Vanilla Ice who notes that Zumba is "'like MTV was back in the day.'"

The rise of these "boutique fitness classes," Rosman argues, has helped the growth of the music business as well. Rosman offers several other examples including a "March Music Madness" competition at Gold's Gym and Flywheel Sports whose "music strategy for its indoor cycling classes" was planned before the studio opened in New York. The songs compiled for Flywheel clients can be heard in spinning studios in "Chicago, Seattle and Dubai" and artists pitch Flywheel regularly to have their music included. Rosman also notes that instructors often post their playlists and that some clubs like SoulCycle forbid this sharing of lists, arguing that music is one of the reasons people come to the classes. SoulCycle hopes to cut their own deal, which speaks to the nature of music and copyright protection and the danger to individual instructors who do not have the resources that corporations do.

In an industry that is tightly controlled by copyright, music can be a dangerous tool to play with. Many certification programs absorb the cost of copyrights, selling it as a part of the choreography package and limiting use to its trained instructors. Some music providers like 32mix.com sell only to instructors. In Australia, fitness studios and individual instructors (and anyone using music in commercial settings) are expected to pay fees for using music during classes. The resources needed to enforce such are unwieldy; it seems impossible to enforce in such an unregulated system. Perhaps this is one of the reasons why such copyright laws are contested. Ben Eltham writes in "The Copyright Cops": "In a decision handed down in May, the Copyright Tribunal ruled that gyms and fitness centres [sic] will have to pay $15 for each class, or $1 per attendee of each class, for the use of the music, up from around $1 a class previously, with a cap of $2654 a year. Representatives of the industry are now appealing that decision." Exercise businesses pay for music because they have to; they make a profit off of the music that accompanies their workouts, particularly those forms of fitness that rely upon music for their choreography. If I had to pay copyright fees on top of the many other expenses I shoulder as a fitness instructor, or if the YMCA had to pay the kinds of fees Eltham discusses, the use of music that is familiar and holds the potential for creativity and empowerment would be off limits to me. Not only would I, and the participants in my classes suffer, so would the artists. As Rosman shows, the music played in classes is just another way to expose people to new music. If you play it, they will come and they will buy it.

Having choice over music is an important tool in an instructor's toolbox, particularly when we want to create an atmosphere in class toward empowerment and enjoyment. I have been able to reconnect with my teenage love of pop music as songs by Britney Spears, Lady Gaga, Katy Perry, Shakira, the Black Eyed Peas, and Rihanna are often much more simple to choreograph —

and are often more fun for participants who recognize these artists and are familiar with the song. But I also include artists who rarely, if ever, appear in mixer music or manufactured fitness programs like: Ani diFranco, Tracey Chapman, M.I.A., Spearhead, Santigold, Blackilicious, The Coup, Nas, Lupe Fiasco, Eminem, Gnarles Barkley, Janelle Monáe, The Yeah Yeah Yeahs, and The Gorillaz. Ultimately, I use music that speaks to me in some way, music I enjoy politically or aesthetically. I give myself permission to play with music and movement — to work with music that would otherwise offend and make it something different. There is something deeper to my music selection as well.

As someone whose musical focus has always been on the lyrics, the music is more carnal to me — a territory I do not understand with the same clarity with which I understand the words. Thus the music I hear — whether a song from my personal collection of the latest hits being overplayed — when the music hits ... it implants itself in my brain and grows through my body. I cannot memorize or remember well most anything; but I have a catalog of dozens, even hundreds, of songs and moves on file in my brain. I mix and remix, plan and improvise. It is a powerful and empowering process and part of my toolbox.

* * *

Feminist fitness pedagogy and methodology for group fitness requires a tool box. As fitness instructors we compose a toolbox of moves, approaches, chunks of choreography, songs, successful workouts, modifications — all of which we stock through trainings and other resources like magazines, but more through observation of other instructors (in DVDs and online videos) and modification based upon our application of these tools. As academics we also have a toolbox — of theories, critiques, politics, observations, and applications — and in both settings we use the tools that are best fitted for the work we are doing. In fitness, these methods lend themselves to cross-training; in academia, to interdisciplinarity.

While interdisciplinary endeavors are alive and well in many educational institutions (Strober 5) — and this approach can be instrumental in professional fields like science and medicine, education, business, and social work as well as the social sciences and humanities (Lattuca 3) — this unknown territory can be frightening to some of us. Disciplinary boundaries are still tightly drawn in some spaces. We don't often have a reason to step outside of our disciplinary boundaries; we specialize, dig deeper, and these foci influence our research and teaching interests.[4] Bonnie Thornton Dill and Ruth Enid

Zambrana explain that "traditional disciplinary boundaries and the compartmentalization and fixity of ideas are challenged by these emerging interdisciplinary fields [which are] identifying new issues, new forms, and new ways of viewing" humanity and social life (2). As a scholar of American Studies and Women's Studies interdisciplinarity is inherent to the work I do in and out of the classroom, and yet the particulars of theory and method in these areas are still contested. Interdisciplines like women's studies and American studies suffer, Lisa Lattuca argues, "not only from a reputation for superficiality, but from the unfamiliar and unsettling effects of its ideas" (4).

Interdisciplinarity is confused with multidisciplinarity and transdisciplinarity. It is understood and practiced differently depending upon the individuals involved and the disciplinary and interdisciplinary contexts in which they work. It is also flexible depending upon the object/subject of study.[5] This slippery quality is, perhaps, part of what people fear about interdisciplinary programs and curricula. When we are not sure what box to put it into, and if there is no box that has the proper dimensions, the subject can become something to ignore or muddle through or contest. But we cannot afford to ignore interdisciplinarity; to contest it is futile. As Allen Repko notes, there is "growing recognition that [interdisciplinarity] is needed to answer complex questions, solve complex problems, and gain coherent understanding of complex issues that are increasingly beyond the ability of any single discipline...." (3). American fitness is full of complex issues, questions, and problems.

In both academic and fitness settings we can use tools from both fitness and academic toolboxes. We can increase our pleasure and power as we study feminist movement. We can increase our critical prowess as we get down. We should also work more diligently to make such toolboxes available to fitness participants and members of our communities. We can move our bodies and our minds. We can transform ourselves and our world with these tools ... in theory and in movement.

Academic Perspectives on Fitness, Feminist Foundations

"Up until now, the gym simply has been where I go at the end of my work and writing days and also during my weekends. As I turn my attention to theorizing this experience, the muscle work and the community, I've entered a body of feminist critique that addresses women and sport, women and fitness, and women and recreation. The essays and poems brought together in this book begin to describe an experience of community and connection that women build and have built

through their bodies and the often happy work of keeping them in motion."
        — Jo Malin, Introduction to *My Life at the Gym* (5)

Like Malin, I have recently turned to the work of theorizing my gym experience. For most of my academic life I was unfamiliar with the scholarly geography of fitness, in part because the bulk of work was done in the sciences. I was afraid to look much further because I did not want to pull my focus away from the more "serious" scholarly pursuits I was learning about in my M.A. and Ph.D. programs. Fitness seemed like it would be a distraction from the cultural and critical theory that defined my programs. I dabbled but I did not go too deep as there were plenty of demands on my time and attention. I had not only a full-time load academically, I also had a part-time load teaching fitness. Balancing these two meant that fitness had to support, not distract from academia.

Especially in recent years, fitness is becoming a serious academic pursuit in areas outside of exercise sciences where fitness got serious in the mid to late 20th century. As the editors of *Women and Exercise* explain, "through mainly qualitative examinations, these researchers have focused on the health benefits of exercise" (Kennedy and Markula 1). One such example is *Women and Exercise: Physiology and Sports Medicine* (1994) which provides a "blend of basic and clinical science ... providing comprehensive coverage for both researchers and clinicians" (vii). Contributors to this volume, the editors note, "have shared their vast experience in a valuable composite of science and art" (vii). However, the past decades have produced a number of academic resources that explore fitness in a variety of incarnations. In her excellent introduction to *Women, Sport, Society: Further Reflections, Reaffirming Mary Wollstonecraft*, Roberta J. Park details developments in fitness-related scholarship and notes that "the tendency on the part of many scholars [in the 1960s and 70s] had been to deal mostly with theoretical or abstract conceptions of 'the body' and to try to interpret what these presumably have meant" (3). She notes the differences between science and social science. Science is about "physics and chemistry" and social science concerns itself with a "'neutral surface or landscape on which a social symbolism is imprinted'" (3).[6]

In the sciences, fitness is broken down into myriad areas and methods of exploration. As William J. Broad explains: "The academic world has a number of research fields that lavish attention on questions of fitness. The disciplines include biomechanics, kinesiology, exercise physiology, nutrition, physical therapy, and sports medicine, among others.... Major universities have whole departments that do nothing but conduct fitness studies and publish the results in dozens of specialty journals...." (48–9). All of these studies, as diverse as they are, approach fitness from a scientific viewpoint and disciplinary segregation means that these studies are often uninformed by other academic fields. Likewise, developments in the social sciences or humanities might not take into account the biological aspects of academic studies of fitness. Disciplinary segregation means that with each field working toward its particular goals, with its particular tools, particular accounts are created. And there is scholarly value in this arrangement as much as there is a missing big picture of what "fitness" is. We might consider that in the humanities, the body is a text to be read and interpreted from a variety of angles and in the arts the body might be a tool, a creative medium, or even a canvas. As an art, however, the social and cultural relevance of fitness becomes embodied and abstracted. These disciplinary perspectives provide different, complementary ways of thinking about fitness. We need to develop and connect the nets that we cast when we research and write about — and practice — fitness.

* * *

Not surprisingly, much of the academic work that has been done surrounding women and fitness outside the sciences, comes from a feminist perspective. Since women's studies and the social sciences are concerned with representations of the body, it makes sense that we would find some concern with fitness and health as well. But, just because a work is about women does not mean it is inherently feminist, even though there are many different feminist lenses that we can use to understand fitness. Some feminist fitness forms are influenced by power feminism — get big and kick ass! Others by feminist psychology or philosophy. Some by more radical analyses — equality, reformist, revolutionary.

My Life at the Gym makes important feminist contributions to academic considerations of fitness and different ways of thinking about fitness. Toward the end of her introduction Jo Malin describes her project:

> *My Life at the Gym* brings together women's narratives, meaningful life narratives that need to be heard as part of a feminist project to describe and deconstruct the lives of women today. Scholars from the humanities, education, law, and women's and literary theory, as well as poets, writers, and visual artists, have sought and are finding meaning and community in diverse sites of physical movement and fitness: gyms, dance studios, skating rinks, boxing rings, and more. Their contributions are multidimensional and diverse and can speak to many other women who seek health and long life in the twenty-first century [14].

To have a group of scholars confessing and critiquing, explaining and exploring the impacts of various kinds of fitness activities in their lives and their work, is a powerful contribution to feminist studies and to academic studies of fitness more generally. The diversity of disciplines and activities represented speak to the diversity of women's fitness experiences and the ways in which fitness can bring together women across difference. The works in this book are critical, but they are also creative, academic, and personal.

While *Women, Sport, Society: Further Reflections, Reaffirming Mary Wollstonecraft* makes important contributions to the larger field of sports, health, and physical education, and while *My Life at the Gym* offers a more personal and introspective exploration of women's fitness, *Women and Exercise: The Body, Health, and Consumerism* focuses on fitness-related issues and takes a more traditional social science feminist approach. It is also heavily imbued with a social sciences approach as each chapter follows the same general outline of introduction, theoretical framework, methodology, application, and conclusion. This rigid structure is important to legitimate scholarly studies of women and exercise within the academy, particularly since several contributors use their personal involvement in a particular fitness culture as evidence to be evaluated academically.

Women and Exercise postulates its purpose as "contributing to [the] growing body of literature that examines the *socio-cultural aspects* of women's exercise" (Kennedy and Markula 1; my emphasis). Editors, Pirkko Markula and Eileen Kennedy provide an extensive overview of socio-cultural scholarship surrounding women and exercise in their introduction, "Beyond Binaries: Contemporary Approaches to Women and Exercise." They argue that "media representations" and "lived experiences" have constituted the bulk of the socio-cultural work regarding fitness, with the former dominating the field and the latter beginning to grow. Further, these foci have "resulted in a series of binaries that, rightly or wrongly, tend to characterize feminist research in fitness" (1). Their introduction then goes on to closely detail previous findings related to women and exercise that illustrate these binaries and provide an intricate map of the socio-cultural academic perspective on fitness.

Tara Brabazon's 2006 article in *Australian Feminist Studies*, "Fitness Is a Feminist Issue" gives us a solid basis from which to study fitness through a critical feminist lens. In this work, Brabazon lays the foundation for considering a number of important aspects of fitness and then begins to tease out the ways in which feminism can make interventions in fitness. She explains, "I often argue that aerobics is an important intervention in the masculine modalities of sport, providing a pleasurable site for community building among women. Much feminist literature disagrees with me. The confluence between exercise and diet, aerobics and eating disorders, punctuates the scholarship" (65). We can't out-run these problems, but they don't need to define

our fitness foci. Her article goes on to consider these important and problematic confluences arguing that "now is the time to unravel this tight bundle
of woman/self/food/exercise/addiction" (78). *Women and Fitness in American
Culture* works toward these ends.

* * *

In academia, few studies of fitness take up issues of race, ethnicity, or
nationality, and even less often, issues of whiteness. Some scientific studies
that focus on particular populations will examine the health or fitness of, for
instance, middle-aged black women or Mexican children. But such studies
work from a position of assumptions about race that may be uncritical and
reflects the impacts of socio-economic conditions rather than biological realities or even social constructions. For instance, an article on the website Medical News Today, details a study "led by Amy J. McMichael, M.D., [that]
found that complications of hair care is the main reason why African-American
women don't exercise as much as they'd like to." This brief, informative article
mostly quotes McMichael regarding the findings of the study, concluding that
"'we have to figure out better ways to address this issue.'" Even so, this article
elicited several comments about its truth or absurdity including one who
wrote the first comment: "either begin publishing stories about Caucasian
women avoiding eating to compete with one another for male attention, or
stop this racism disguised as 'medical' reporting." The charge of racism often
functions to ramp up (or shut down) conversation. Here, the comment is
taken up with a certain amount of lucidity. One commenter writes, "I implore
those of you who wish to criticize or censure this article to hold back, and
accept a fact. Denial and paranoia never got anybody anywhere." Another
identifies herself as a health professional and writes, "And the fake nails and
the fake hair is just a way of making herself look good on the outside, even
though many of these women are truly miserable with their weight and are
overwhelmed as to what will truly make a difference." In this brief conversation, about an even briefer article, those who want to go deeper — to consider
and challenge the social construction of beauty and the importance of hair
to constructs of beauty — engage in examining the truths that this article
reveals while still keeping an eye on the larger structural influences.[7]

Brabazon makes important connections in her work between socioeconomic class and racial and ethnic identities in relation to ideas about fitness.
She notes that "anxiety of the obesity 'epidemic' is part of a long-term surveillance of working-class work and leisure" (70). She also notes that in the
U.K. "Black Caribbean and British Asian women particularly, and lower socio-

economic groups more generally, 'suffer' through higher rates of obesity" (71). These trends are similar in the U.S. and while some obesity trends are linked with higher rates of consumption, enabled by a higher socioeconomic class, the issues of poor food, poor support systems, inadequate health care, and other factors mean that poverty and obesity are also linked. Thus, Brabazon argues that it is important for "feminist theorists of sport to recognise [sic] the classed and raced nature of food, health and leisure, but also to carefully differentiate the 'problems' of fatness and fitness" (71).

Sharon Wray begins important work in the direction of radical reconsideration of race in her chapter from *Women and Exercise*, "The Significance of Western Health Promotion Discourse for Older Women from Diverse Ethnic Backgrounds." Wray frames her work through some discussion of problematic multicultural approaches to health promotion like "celebratory inclusion" (163). While her findings and framings are specific to the U.K., they have relevance to similar approaches in the U.S. Both cultures focus on the idea that individuals are in control of their bodies, and thus have personal responsibility regarding their health and physical appearance and abilities. And, most importantly, "structural and material causes of ill health, such as poverty, sexism and racism, tend to be underplayed" (161). An individual's poor fitness is always attributed to her failings, not to the failings of a culture that has structured inequalities built right into the system. Further, as bell hooks argues, "people of color, especially poor people of color, have deep concerns about living well, but they simply lack the resources to focus on health issues. Instead, day-to-day survival is paramount" (*Homegrown* 141). These few examples start a larger conversation about the ways in which race, generally, and whiteness, specifically, are deeply embedded in our mainstream American understandings of fitness.

* * *

All of these works inform my work in this book; however, academic analyses, particularly when laden with theoretical jargon, are limited and limiting to an understanding of fitness in its fullness. I try to translate these ideas for a wider public discussion. I think about the people who work out with me. For many, such academic discussions would be off their radars and out of their comfort zones. Feminist examinations of fitness continue to range from oppressive to empowering readings. These examinations also tend to hover around issues of the body — as a site of oppression and negotiation.[8] The work, then, falls to feminists — in and out of the gym — to continue to understand and illuminate fitness experiences and to develop feminist fitness theory, methodology, and pedagogy. Kennedy and Markula offer an interesting and important perspective in their introduction to *Women and Exercise*. They argue that "feminist researchers" who also "act as fitness instructors" can use "their attempts to negotiate the conflicting and partial understandings of health and fitness in their own exercise classes and their efforts to transcend the current discourses" to "form an aspect of feminist transformative agenda for social change" (21). This is an agenda I explore and expand throughout this book.

Repeat to the Left

Leotards and legwarmers.
I only knew you through my mother's workout record,
Something I didn't really understand
But would sometimes mimic —
you and my mother —
Repeat to the left and to the right.

I didn't know about "Hanoi Jane"
Or the hatred that some men
of a certain generation
Harbored.
I didn't care about politics
When I knew you through
Striped leotards and legwarmers.

When I cared about politics,
I learned about yours
Explored through penetration
Of enemy lines,
posed/poised
on anti-aircraft machinery,
pushed/pressed
to defend your worth.
And for the record
I defend you,
On/for feminist principles.

I didn't know about Barbarella
(or June or Cat or Gloria or Bree or Chelsea
or any of your other faces).
We were only recently introduced
At a conference where I learned
That Barbarella's face (your face)
Was the first face of female orgasm
Seen on film.

When I cared about female orgasm
I happened to learn about yours (hers),

Achieved without penetration,
Without a man,
In a funky 1968 flick,
Only a glimmer
Of your feminist legacy.

An image of
Orgasmic fitness, rebel politics,
Feminist activism,
For a person I can only piece together
Through incomplete understandings,
Past and present,
Public and private,
Political and personal.
You "paid heavily" and compromised —
Still you endured,
Moving millions.

You resonate —
Your many faces, many stages, many transformations —
Burned into my mind and body,
A fire in my spirit,
A rhythm in
Tank top and yoga pants.

1968: Revolutions

"Aerobics: The word that changed the world."
"Aerobics is a movement filled with people who read a book and followed a plan that changed their life. Aerobics is as important and relevant today as the day it was born in 1968."

— Cooper Aerobics website

In the academic fields in which I teach, the year 1968 has special significance. It is a marker of revolution, of change and of idealistic hope. It is a year when power seems like it could be differently dispersed. It is a year of violent oppressions and fearless uprisings. It is the year that Dr. Martin Luther King, Jr. and Senator Robert F. Kennedy were assassinated. It is the year that feminists protested against the Miss America Beauty Contest, emblazoning the "bra burners" into the popular imagination. Jane Fonda starred as Barbarella, claiming women's sexuality. Abbie Hoffman's Yippies demonstrated at the Chicago Democratic National Convention with a "Festival of Life." Tommie Smith and John Carlos "disrupted" the Olympic Games by performing the black power salute during their medal ceremony. 1968 is a year that students in the U.S. and around the world protested against war, racism, and other oppressions. It is a year that embodies revolution.

It is also the year that Kenneth H. Cooper's book *Aerobics* was published. This accessible, encouraging, informative (if also a bit pedantic) international best-seller is credited with beginning a revolutionary fitness movement in America and around the world. Cooper's work in *Aerobics* grew from the work he did with the Air Force and NASA in the mid–60s and has also created a platform for his life's work. As I have noted, before Cooper's work, "fitness" was defined by doctors as "freedom from disease" and *Aerobics* was foundational in establishing fitness as an important endeavor for American's physical, and to a lesser extent mental, health. The media and the medical establishment were both weary of this new phenomenon and Cooper had to defend his research (Bass). Cooper sold the idea of "aerobics," at least in part, based upon the measureable benefits he observed when working with members of the Air Force. His approach to fitness is pure science as it concerns itself with health and provides readers with a measureable strategy with specific goals. And the preface by a Senator and introduction by a Lt. General give the book legitimacy and a solid American context.

Despite these persuasive factors, Cooper's research and suggestions were not immediately accepted. As long-time columnist for *Muscle & Fitness*, Clarence Bass, explains in his article about Cooper and the 40th anniversary of *Aerobics*, Cooper had to fight a "battle" with the "medical establishment" and the media. He recounts Cooper's writing about Barbara Walters's skepticism, which ended with his being booked on the *Today Show*. And when he moved his family to Dallas to open a "private preventative medical practice.... The Dallas County Medical Society tried to shut him down." Of this battle, Cooper says, "'Many people don't realize the challenges I've faced. Aerobics and preventive medicine haven't always been popular,' says Cooper. 'I persevered through it all because I knew that a healthy life means a long and productive life" (Bass). However, these "challenges" are hardly those faced by people with other revolutionary ideas in 1968. Cooper's battle was fought with his state-sanctioned research which, ultimately, won him the war.

In 1970 he opened the Cooper Institute for Aerobic research (later the Cooper Institute) and "In 1986, Dr. Cooper submitted the definition of *Aerobics* to the *Oxford English Dictionary*" (Bass). The definition reads, "Method of physical exercise for producing beneficial changes in the respiratory and circulatory systems by activities which require meeting a modest increase in oxygen intake and so can be maintained" (Cooper Aerobics). As William J. Broad notes in the *Science of Yoga*, before Cooper this concept of aerobics in relation to human fitness "was long obscure" (53) and Cooper's findings led to "a number of scientific inquiries that examined what aerobic exercise could do not only for athletics but health. The results were dramatic" (54). American fitness would never be the same; *Aerobics* did, in fact, spur a kind of revolution in fitness and our approaches to fitness have certainly changed, even if the problems (poor health and lack of physical activity) that led to our need for a better definition of fitness, and a better process for achieving it, remain.

Cooper's work has inspired countless individuals' fitness pursuits and he has continued to be a presence and visionary in the world of fitness. Over the past 40 years Cooper has expanded his work in fitness from "aerobics" to include other aspects like strength-training, spirituality, and overall well-being. His nonprofit Cooper Institute has expanded into the online space Cooper Aerobics and he has published more than 20 books since *Aerobics*, including: *Faith-Based Fitness: The Medical Program That Uses Spiritual Motivation to Achieve Maximum Health and Add Years to Your Life* and *Regaining the Power of Youth at Any Age: Startling New Evidence from the Doctor Who Brought Us Aerobics*. Cooper's books build upon one another and have expanded the idea of aerobics to women and children specifically and has also addressed a wider range of fitness concerns. As Bass points out, Cooper has turned his attention to wellness, which includes: "weight control, good nutrition, proper supplementation, not smoking, limiting alcohol, controlling stress, and periodic medical and fitness exams."

Cooper and his son, Tyler, have not simply created a revolution in fitness, they have also created an extensive family business, expanding the Cooper Institute and creating the Cooper Aerobics corporation which includes eight health and wellness companies and provides products and services, classes and certifications, to individuals and businesses. The Cooper Clinic, Cooper Fitness Center, Cooper Guest Lodge, Cooper Wellness, Cooper Concepts, Inc. (which oversees the creation to distribution of Cooper Complete Nutritional Supplements), Cooper Spa, Cooper Weight Loss, and Cooper Corporate Solutions form a kind of Cooper fitness empire. Ironically, Cooper's empire is not a far stretch from the solution that he poses in the concluding pages of *Aerobics*. Cooper calls for more attention to coordination of research efforts and a "more sophisticated approach" (163). Both important developments that have come to fruition, but his "more serious complaint is directed at the American attitude in general toward exercise." He continues, "with the great majority of the population in a deconditioned state, something obviously is wrong" (163). His "more sophisticated approach" is a solution modeled after Europe, setting up "rehabilitation camps" for the deconditioned so that they might become more productive workers, miss less work, and retire later in life. The only thing Cooper sees that could be "wrong" with this is that "Americans generally hate being told what to do" (164). We might imagine why "rehabilitation camps" weren't such a good idea in 1968, in part based upon the racialized assumptions and goals that underlie the "unfit" and "deconditioned" masses in America. Yet, Cooper has realized the American version of this dream.

Cooper's developments in fitness represent a "revolution" in "aerobics," and ultimately health and fitness, as much as they represent an example of successful American capitalist endeavors and the sanction of American institutional authority. His is a success story that is undergirded by the authority that he holds as a result of his status. As a doctor, we must accept his authority when it comes to matters of health. Since his research was funded and backed by the U.S. government, and collected and synthesized based upon the physical fitness pursuits of our military men (and a very few women), he holds the status and authority that come with these American institutions. And as a white man, his other identities are only strengthened in their authority. His empire is not simply built upon his revolutionary views of fitness and the importance and impact of his work; it is also built upon the assumptions that come from his place of authority in our culture.

It feels ironic, but is, perhaps, only coincidental that these two seemingly separate interests of mine — social justice and fitness — should coincide with this marker of the year 1968. Certainly fitness has been shaped by many of the same forces that have also shaped the nature of politics — the fitness industry is driven by the same economic system that drives corrupt politicians and businessmen. The use of the fitness industry to make women and men feel bad about their bodies, to get us to consume any number of products and services toward an ideal body, is like the use of other industries to undermine people's confidences and waste their time on distractions from political change. And this is one of the cultural contradictions of contemporary revolutionary movement and why mind/body transformations are important revolutionary tools.

Social Justice and Academia's Secret Life

"Suddenly I had the freedom to think, to reflect. I thought that aspiring to be happy was as valid a goal as making a revolution; without the wisdom to forge my own happiness, how could I presume to save the world?... (344)
I know that the obsession to redeem humanity can be just as dangerous as the fanaticism I see in the faces of those who dedicate themselves to perfect bodies, pure, unadulterated food, and the quest for immortality. I try to think that each and every one of us is responsible for finding meaning and purpose in life, and that it's arrogant to think that my solution is better than the rest. On the other hand, I don't think anyone could ever convince me that the kind of pleasure that

begins and ends in oneself can even remotely be compared to the exaltation and joy that comes from joining others in the effort to change the world." (366–7)

— Gioconda Belli, *The Country Under My Skin: A Memoir of Love and War*

"The empowerment fantasies on offer [by Oprah, for instance, and the media more generally] are personal, not collective, they are about 'me,' not about making things better for all girls and women. In fact, if I come to feel, like, really empowered, having written in my journal while drinking herb tea after having done my yoga, wouldn't I be so at peace, so blissed out, that I'd be completely happy with exactly the way things are?" (150)

— Susan J. Douglas from *The Rise of Enlightened Sexism: How Pop Culture Took Us from Girl Power to Girls Gone Wild*

"Welcome to a new era where we're not going to apologize for what we've earned the right to be. The ones with "FUCK YOU" in our DNA will show the world a fiercely naked, feral and cornered kind of love ... that doesn't sit passively on yoga mats with enlightened wedgies, thinking trademarked thoughts, and assuming that's enough to change the world."

— Erika Lopez, *The Girl Must Die: A Monster Girl Memoir*

"The contributors in this collection, many of whom are academics and writers, describe ways in which inclusion of regular physical exercise in their otherwise cerebral lives is enriching and very basic to their health and identities as aware feminists. They have also found a sense of community...."

— Jo Malin, Introduction to *My Life at the Gym*

These epigraphs reflect the kinds of attitude that some academics have toward "fitness"— the idea as well as the practice. Belli's revelation that "aspiring to be happy was as valid a goal as making a revolution" might be seen as arrogant and superficial, but this belief comes, in part, from her observations of "fanaticism" and the effects that this state of mind might have on revolutionaries. She compares this fanaticism to "those who dedicate themselves to perfect bodies, pure, unadulterated food, and the quest for immortality"; this fanaticism, this goal of perfection, is not "fitness" and is not a balanced approach to life, body, or revolution. In this kind of fanaticism there is not room for happiness, even the happiness that Belli describes: "the exaltation and joy that comes from joining others in the effort to change the world." Fitness makes room for the mind, enhances the work of the mind. This is at least partly a result of stress relief and happiness endorphins. Those of us who exercise regularly know this or, rather, we *feel* this.[9] By making room for happiness — for a fitness of body and mind — we are also making ourselves more valuable for the causes that we care about passionately. Both Belli and Douglas assume an either/or stance; neither happiness nor social change are compatible with pursuits of physical fitness. And Lopez and Douglas associate yoga with distraction from change rather than as a tool toward transformation. But Malin redefines physical exercise as "enriching and very basic." Happiness is, after all, a personal benefit as much as it can be a collective benefit.

* * *

There are certainly many differences and variations between and among the work of social justice, social service, and service in the realm of academics. In my academic work, not only is service a requirement of the job description, but the impetus to continue to serve — the students, the campus, the academic unit, and the community — is derived from my academis work.[10] Despite the presence of fitness in my life, I continue to find little balance in my all-consuming life in academia. This work is stressful, demanding. I love it. Fitness makes this work possible. It inserts some very needed time to move and to think in different ways and to avoid thinking about the millions of things to do, papers to grade, events to plan, students and colleagues and prospectives to call, to write. I devote huge chunks of time to teaching, advising, grading, planning, organizing, writing, researching, reading, meeting, sorting, filling out paperwork, answering emails, managing crises, encouraging and listening to my students and colleagues, etc.... And our lives are filled with work and then children and lives and pets and family and ... the gym ... or the trails, or the studio, or.... We spread ourselves thin and often devote ourselves to our students and to our institution. Our work is extremely rewarding, and we can see the positive effects of our work at least as much as we are confronted by students' struggles, budget crises, negotiations, meeting after meeting, and the shrinking employment opportunities we are preparing our students to meet.

Many of my professors, mentors, colleagues, advisors, students, and staff have regular workout routines. The activities that compose fitness vary for all of them. And, yet, fitness is a difficult thing to work into our daily/weekly routines. Some of us know the importance and fail to make the time and some of us simply don't know, or ignore, the detrimental effects of not having a physical release, a time for the body to be energized and the mind to be cleared. Perhaps a lack of an interest or focus on fitness is an issue of time: we have a lot of duties and we all (most) work really hard. Surely fitness detracts from these serious, professional duties. Perhaps it is an issue of perception. We are all about the mind. To admit to the pursuits of the body would be to admit to vanity, to a desire to look good. Perhaps a desire to please the patriarchy. This is certainly the idea we get from Susan Douglas's snarky and flippant reference to yoga if not from the image on the cover of her book — a woman turned away from the camera, sporting a white tank top and pristine bubblegum-pink boxing gloves (in a non-fighting pose). She implies that one's personal pursuits of empowerment must somehow be at odds with empowerment for all women and girls; she reinforces a binary that underscores academia's relationship with fitness. She also illustrates an ignorance shattered by feminist scholars who address fitness and empowerment in their work.

* * *

The connections between fitness and activism might also have more potential for social change and social justice as Jaime Schultz explores in her article, "The Physical is Political: Women's Suffrage, Pilgrim Hikes and the Public Sphere." In this piece she explores the women's suffrage movement and the concept of "physical activism": "the articulation of physical activity and political activism — striking simultaneous blows to the *myths* of women's *physical and political inferiority*" (29; my emphasis). She argues that "while the political is the impetus for human movement, the physical is no less important; indeed, the act would lack the same resonance if the statement had been expressed in any other way" (31). Schultz's exploration of physical activism is not so much concerned with, for instance, fund-raising "thons" like those for breast cancer or Alzheimer's (a popular mode for socially conscious fitness. Example: the fundraiser); instead, she illustrates the convergence of state violence and protest where women's bodies took the brunt of the state's resistance to women's suffrage. Most Americans don't know the violent, brute force our Suffragette mothers endured.[11] Still, these are the more familiar uses of the body — the sacrifice of one's body through civil disobedience or protest, the willingness to endure pain or even death for one's cause.

But Schultz also examines protest actions, "spectacles" like Pilgrim Hikes where women were able to "[debunk] the myth of female frailty that had been used to argue against their enfranchisement" (31), draw attention to women's struggles, and, make important political statements. For instance, a 1912 letter to *Woman's Journal* by one Pilgrim Hike participant made the case that their hike was nothing compared to the working conditions of American women and, thus, "demonstrated the ways in which physical expressions might draw attention to multiple socio-political causes of the day" (40). Here, the physical exertion of the hike drew attention to the physical discrimination of women's labor. While it might be easy to imagine the ways in which the body figures into movements like the U.S. Civil Rights movement, "of all the tools available to groups and individuals in a given society, the body seems the most fundamental and perhaps the most underestimated possibility for enacting change" (46). In other words, the body has more potential in movement than it does in the act of sitting still, literally and figuratively. It is real while it is also symbolic. Schultz introduces the concept of "physical activism" as a way of better understanding the role and potential of the body. And if the body is to be a tool in "corporeal action" (46), it must be kept ready for action.

Tara Brabazon introduces what is, perhaps, one of the most important ideas linking fitness and social justice. She argues that "the right to organised [sic], productive and publicly funded fitness progammes [sic] is a new imperative for social justice, class consciousness and agency. Such an attention to leisure, fitness and sport allows a remapping of social structures" (70). She discusses some of the arguments that people make against publicly funded fitness programs that pay for shoes, for instance, and other costs associated with fitness. Some such arguments are commonplace in a variety of spheres; why should we pay for fitness when we could be paying for cancer screenings or why pay for food stamps when people are obese. "Preventative medicine — through fitness — is not a waste of resources" (71), Brabazon argues. Promoting fitness is, then, one way of reducing future costs to the state. But this bigger picture is not always convincing, especially where neo-conservative politics reign and the power of the individual is assumed to be enough to create change.

The focus on the individual is one of the challenges that confuses yoga's dimensions of service and community. *21st Century Yoga: Culture, Politics, and Practice* considers several discussions of yoga's potential and to impact people toward social responsibility and community support. Matthew Remski describes yoga's current state as "a cultural adolescent" that "wants self-expression and constant redefinition. Today, yoga is more about identity than it is about service" (111). Even as yoga shifts its cultural foot-hold, individuals and groups recognize its uses toward transformation. Some of these may border on romanticism. Michael Stone, for instance, explores the possibilities born of imagination and social movement (specifically the Occupy movement) and also argues that "we need to slow down and return to values of relationality and interdependence. This is where yoga comes in. Yoga teaches us that we are much happier when we serve others" (160). As true as the sentiment may be for many individuals, just as yoga is no panacea for health, it is certainly not a magical gateway to activism and social and cultural transformation. Be Scofield cautions that "engaging in meditation or yoga is no guarantee of distancing oneself from the values, morals, or institutions that shape the surrounding society" (135). In fact, "they can also be consciously or unconsciously used to support the status quo" (135).

The social, cultural, and economic environment of the status quo is hostile to the idea of fitness as transformative. As Brabazon argues, in a "climate where the only site of personal control is the body. The desire for social change is displaced through a goal of personal transformation" (73). We adhere to a fitness version of the bootstraps theory even though we know that American myths of meritocracy have never held weight. These are just some of the reasons why, Brabazon argues, "fitness can and should be used by feminists to further the social, political and collectivist struggles" (75). Like the women "who occupy the city streets...," we are "not temporarily passing through...." We are here, grounded.

* * *

One of the women famous for her occupation of the city streets, is activist, political prisoner, and radical professor Angela Davis. Founder of Critical Resistance, an organization that works to abolish prisons, Angela Davis is the last person I would expect to see chained to a treadmill. But, at a talk that Angela Davis gave at a nearby private college in 2010, she described a networking session that she engaged in at the gym before a conference. Instantly my attention was peaked. Here is Angela Davis mentioning — in public, in a serious academic setting — that she works out. That she spends time on a *piece of cardio equipment.*[12] If Angela Davis can admit this, then why am I so shy about my life in fitness? Fitness is not a regime that needs to be upheld as a means to maintain the aging body any more than it is a means to a mass-media-approved body; it is not counter to or even simply complementary to our lives outside of the gym. Fitness is an integrated part of a whole person, a person strong enough, balanced enough, to continually face the monsters inside of us and all around us.

Fitness is not about "sit[ting] passively on yoga mats with enlightened wedgies"; the mind/body connection requires much more than passivity but it also requires that we do not simply retreat within ourselves — our own minds and bodies. We might not strive to "save" the world. We might strive to change the world, or a part of the world. We might just need the stamina — the mental and physical strength — to get through the long days devoted to others.[13] In conversation with Amalia Mesa-Bains in *Homegrown*, bell hooks reminds us that "broad coalitions can be built around" issues like health and housing. She argues, "this is what I call practical activism — an activism that's connected to where you live, and to the vision of being homegrown" (141). It takes a kind of fitness of the mind and body to be able to give of ourselves and still have enough to renew this giving, to be "homegrown" in our vision and approach.

THREE

Toward a Theory of Feminist Fitness

Women and Fitness, Igniting Feminist Foundations

"In her 1792 treatise A Vindication of the Rights of Woman, Mary Wollstonecraft proclaimed that when girls were allowed to take the same exercise as boys the fiction of the 'natural superiority of man' would be exposed. A century later, as growing numbers of women began engaging in sports and achieving a place of distinction in the profession of physical education, her assertion became a reality."
— Roberta J. Park, "Women as Leaders: What Women Have Attained in and Through the Field of Physical Education" (166)

Mary Wollstonecraft's argument is foundational for studies of women in fitness. Such sentiments have certainly inspired policies like Title IX as well as the early feminist roots in gymnastics, dance, sports, and physical education programs that Park considers. But the kind of practical work that women do in the field of education or through sports have been separated, perhaps even segregated from our understandings of women and fitness. While the wealth of feminist critique concerning body image has touched upon fitness out of necessity, the assumptions that "healthful exercise is unfeminist" (Malin 3) has lead to a rift between *feminist* understandings of fitness and *feminine* understandings of fitness. Feminine understandings keep women in boxes of the perfect body, a focus, on appearance, and a fear of building muscles and strength. Feminist understandings are the antidote to these superficial fitness agendas.

Feminine understanding is rooted in ideas embedded in American consciousness long before Kenneth Cooper described women as comprising a "special group" (56). Cooper's early insights are clear reflections of male dominance and patriarchy's influence on how men saw women's fitness as well as how women saw their own fit bodies. While the studies that supported *Aerobics* were almost exclusively done on men, in his analyses of women's fitness needs Cooper argues in a matter-of-fact tone that women "fall for fads and shortcuts, and spend the time they save on exercising working on their hair or makeup, but they really don't worry about it.... A lot of women miss the point, and I'd be less than honest if I didn't say it's because the American woman is less interested in her health than in her looks" (82–3). If the ingrained cultural assumptions of the 1950s are not obvious in 1968, Cooper goes on to explain that "not so many years ago, women accepted sweat as part of their daily life" (83). Their household chores provided all of the exercise they needed while "today, push-buttons do most of the chores and women spend more time in front of television sets than their sedentary husbands" (83). Cooper's racial and class assumptions are achingly apparent.

The modern conveniences of "push-buttons" mean that chores are not the answer to women's fitness needs; instead, "it has to be some form of aerobic exercise" (84), and then Cooper goes on to detail the "ladylike" activities that might appeal to women including swimming and rope skipping as well as the kinds of sports "easily adaptable to women" (85) like golf, tennis, and skiing. Finally, he notes that women "might notice some change in personality," noting one woman who claimed she was "'not as mean as [she] used to be'" (85). Cooper will "settle for that," implying that his concerns about women's fitness are much less concerns about health than they are concerns about women's superficiality though, to be fair, he does note that he wishes he could write an article for women about exercise and "have them believe every word of it" (82). Women's indifference to exercise is, after all, "one of the great disappointments of [his] career" (82), at least his career up to 1968. But in her 2003 work, in an overview of Kenneth Cooper's *Aerobics*, Gina Kolata notes some of these same observations about Cooper's take on women and yet offers no critique or analysis, simply observation.

The growth of the women's movement in the U.S. is certainly linked to struggling against such patronly sentiments (and the norming of these attitudes about women) as well as to the rise in women's interest in sports and fitness and other pursuits traditionally dominated by men. And yet, as reported by *Women and Exercise* "international studies still report a stubborn gender difference in participation levels — women exercise less than men" (1). Certainly this is due, in part, to the continuing inequality in reproductive labor — the house work and the child care. And it is certainly not unrelated to the ways in which women's bodies are represented in popular culture as objects and with the assumption that beautiful, flawless bodies are naturally fit. Even though we know this is not true, the myth is still powerful. As Kennedy and Markula observe, "in this equation, the responsibility of the healthy looking body is assigned to individual women" (3).[1] And when women bear this responsibility we "leave the societal construction of oppressive *femininity* unchallenged" (3; my emphasis). This focus on the individual speaks to mainstream American values of self-sufficiency and independence. But for women it is also about beauty — that binding "societal construction of oppressive femininity." With feminism, fitness digs below the superficial.[2]

Simply studying women and exercise, sport, health, or fitness, like any other field, does not assume a feminist approach. *My Life at the Gym* and *Women and Exercise* are two academic works that take a "specifically feminist perspective into their analyses of the fit, feminine body" (Kennedy and Markula 1).[3] Throughout this book I unflinchingly take up a feminist lens and agenda concerning the topic of American fitness. Because American fitness takes as its default norm patriarchal ideas and idealized forms, this book assumes that the norm can be better understood by considering fitness from a feminist perspective. Chapter Three focuses specifically on ideas about, and issues related to, feminism. I explore definitions of feminism and fitness and imagine what feminist fitness might look like in theory and on the ground. I consider how we might search for and find feminist incarnations of fitness, individually as well as in community. I attempt to theorize and model feminist fitness — and a melding of the creative and the critical — as well.

Any foray into deepening feminist understanding begins with a shout! A leap toward movement.

The F Word[4]

Designated by "F"
(as if we did not know the whole word)
Feminist and Fuck
Are both *bad words*

You should not call yourself a _____
(and whether a feminist or not)
You should not want to _____

You should not hold political opinions or
Flesh and blood desires

You should not build community or
Break down barriers
Between body and mind

You should not ostracize yourself by
Qualifying yourself for a label (SLUT)
Pursuing carnal knowledge or
Social justice

You should not remember that
Feminists come in a variety of shades
And fuck is also a four-letter word
Used for power and to dis-empower
Through many incarnations

F words are flesh — body & soul
Full of pleasure and passion
Tools for
Fearless
Fucking feminists.

The (Other) F Word

There's the obvious —
the one among the "four letter words"
the other is uncontrollable — movement
that requires its own field
of interpretation.
The first is employed for effect —
anger, frustration, cool.
The other's avoided
because of its implications
or embraced
for its possibilities
or shrugged off
as irrelevant, useless, passé.

And then there's fitness —
an under-the-radar
F word —
a tool of patriarchy
white supremacy
offering superficial gains
(flat abs, tight ass)
rather than embodied transformation.

Bandied about as a means
for "better bodies"/
shucked
for its unattainable image
fearless
fucking feminists
forget fitness
and forge feminist movement.

This F word is
ripe for reclaiming —
a tool toward empowerment,
critical perspective,
transformation.

A way of life —
of balance and flexibility,
strength and endurance,
inspiration and energy.

Connections between
body and mind and
self and community —
Perspective

Employed for effect,
avoided or embraced,
Fitness
enhances the other
F words
in infinite ways.

Feminist Fitness: In Theory and on the Ground

Well-being, self-care, and a whole mind/body approach are at the heart of feminist fitness and its power toward social and cultural transformation. The classic feminist foundation fits well: the personal is political. Fitness manifests itself from within even as it is shaped from without. But feminist fitness goes beyond what advice columns and pseudo research provide. This mode of fitness also challenges what academic studies of fitness can tell us. As Pirkko Markula argues, "despite substantial feminist critique of the fitness industry, there are very few feminist 'interventions' that investigate options for changing the current practices" (61).[5] Markula also suggests that the practices of academics, particularly academic critique, are not often effective in changing the object of study. However, feminist interventions in fitness are taking place outside of academia in a variety of forms.

The term *feminist* is not necessarily present when feminist fitness is on the ground. For instance, Beth Shaw's YogaFit Essence includes "feeling and listening to your body" (14), a technique toward empowerment; and Nia includes the fundamental idea that "Fitness Must Address the Human Being, Not Just the Body" (17), an idea that echoes feminism as well. Jaana Parviainen argues that "the MP [Method Pukisto] can hardly be called a feminist approach, but it includes resistance to the traditional aerobic-oriented fitness culture" (44). Resistance is a start. When brought to individuals and communities, feminist fitness leads to transformations of mind and body that vary, shift, mold, disrupt, balance, and sooth. If brought more consciously — to communities of exercisers as theory — and especially to fitness instructors as method and pedagogy — feminist fitness has the potential to transform individuals, communities, and the bigger picture of American fitness. This question still undergirds explorations of fitness but takes on different terms like "the limitations of dominant definitions of exercise and the ideal body" as well as "how women actively create meanings of their exercise participation" (Kennedy and Markula 21). In other words, the individual struggles against dominant ideals of fitness but can also actively shape their own experiences of exercise.

* * *

The first time I saw the phrase "feminist fitness" was in a 2002 article in *Bitch Magazine: Feminist Response to Popular Culture*. Initially I was afraid to read it. I was in an insecure place — trying to find myself in grad school, trying to figure out where I fit in. I bookmarked it and set it aside. I did not realize how much time had passed before I picked it up again too many years later, when I was ready to think about "feminist fitness." I found an invaluable resource to begin to further develop the fitness ideas that I have discovered mostly through practice. On the ground, feminist fitness is not a foreign concept to those of us who enjoy the many benefits of regular exercise. But, in theory, feminist fitness continues to be in development — formally and informally, in and out of the academy. In terms of group fitness, feminist fitness is less about the content of the class and more about the approach to the class — the instructor's techniques, ideology, and methodology; the music and clothing choices; the physical and social atmosphere created by instructors and participants (and facility owners/directors). But, more widely, a few feminist fitness tenants speak to fitness as a process and a state of being rather than as an end-point or goal.

In her *Bitch Magazine* article, "Beyond the Burn: Toward a Feminist Fitness," Janet Elise Johnson provides a feminist analysis of fitness and begins to imagine what "feminist fitness" might look like. She briefly discusses starting points for a foundation of feminist fitness in theory. She begins with the idea that "feminist fitness is motivated by the goals of women's health and empowerment." While fitness agendas have often been linked to health, and while empowerment is questioned through academic research and promoted in popular fitness magazines in pop feminist forms, the linking of health and empowerment implies a balance of the physical as well as the mental, the health of the body/mind and the empowerment that is complemented by a strong body/mind. A related tenet that Johnson explores is: "Feminist fitness has women's well-being and self-care at its heart." Well-being is bigger than physical health and this tenant is taken up by many mind/body forms of exercise like yoga and Nia, for instance. But self-care is an important aspect of feminism that can intervene in the pressure so many of us feel to be super women. If we don't take care of ourselves, how can we take care of those who rely upon us for care?

Perhaps two of the most important tenants that Johnsons presents are "Feminist Fitness focuses on process" and "Feminist Fitness is a shared experience." So many fitness approaches are based on results: bigger biceps, smaller thighs, better cardio endurance. While these are part of the process, feminist fitness is more of a journey, with stages and education. Further, when we emphasize process over results, we measure progress in other ways — how we feel, what we can do, how we perceive ourselves and others. Process also allows us to always be growing and exploring, to change course when necessary. And process is an experience that can be shared in more healthy and whole ways than physical results can be. While it is easy to see someone's weight loss, it might be more difficult to see her happiness or improved outlook on life. When we are a part of a community we can see the more subtle changes. So, while we might complement and encourage someone who has lost weight, we don't have to focus only on the difference this makes to her appearance. And noticing the deeper changes are a sign of community, a connection that is stronger and more lasting than physical results.

While Johnson's tenants here might seem simple, they are, in fact, part of a revolutionary idea of fitness. Feminist fitness gives us — as instructors and participants — a set of understandings about fitness that we can explore as individuals and communities (and as feminist researchers and critics). But feminist fitness can also give us practical and ideological tools to increase pleasure and power and encourage freedom through movement. These tools connect mind and body, personal and collective. Kristine Newhall, recognizes that many of the problems that feminists have found with "fitness" and the fitness industry "can be mitigated through better instructor training, a commitment to creating a feminist environment, and an overall paradigm shift about group exercise" (68). These three tenants are important in the development of an ideological and practical feminist fitness.

* * *

My first experiences of feminist fitness came through my teaching, and I did not think to call it feminist.[6] When I began training instructors (around the year 2000) I began to develop a set of guidelines and advice that were inspired by a still nascent feminist ideology and sensibility. I taught instructors about the importance of teaching to everyone in the room and being aware of our participants' strengths and weaknesses, as well as our own. I taught not to use phrases like "sit Indian style" and not to encourage participants to work harder in order to burn off that brownie. I chose music that I enjoyed (within the available mixer music) and would omit songs I found to be offensive. I would dress in a way that showed off my body toward emulation of movements but not in a way that showed off my body as if I was putting myself on display. I dressed comfortably. All of these aspects came naturally — from my experience and personality and from what I have learned in and out of fitness. But it took a shift — or many shifts in consciousness to recognize the feminist nature of my work in fitness. Johnson and Newhall have helped me to think about the ways in which my teaching draws upon feminist fitness principles and to continue this development.

Many aspects of feminist fitness I have learned from other instructors, but I have never had a conversation with another instructor where we have talked about feminism or a feminist approach to fitness. In fact, as instructors we don't talk often about our methods, ideologies, or how we approach our work as fitness instructors. Such conversations often revolve around the more mechanical aspects of teaching. Are there three hops or four? How did you teach that move again? So your pattern is.... Many training programs incorporate some version of their brand of fitness ideology, but rarely (never in my experience) would call it such. And I have never been to a training where we have discussed explicitly feminist approaches to fitness, even if the approaches we discussed could be considered "feminist." Thus, I have often wondered why it is that so many fitness instructors incorporate feminist ideas and principles into their teaching and whether they are conscious of the fact that they are doing so. The simplest answer to such a question is to remember that we might consider Feminism to be the most successful and far-reaching social movement of our times, a social movement that has changed and influenced our culture so much that its effects are not always recognized as *feminist*. In fact, many of the changes that feminists have fought for have become norms or have been taken for granted.[7]

The role that fitness instructors play in embodying, modeling, and teaching feminist fitness cannot be understated. Fitness instructors design programs based upon the needs of a wide cross-section of people with varying values, goals, and states of fitness. Because these goals are more general for group exercise instructors than they are for personal trainers, instructors have to offer more open and interpretive versions of movement, more inclusive language, more options for intensity or injury prevention. And there is also the potential to reach more participants than are reached through more tailored individual or small group personal training programs. Thus, one way to bring feminist fitness principles to group exercise, and to fitness programs more generally, is through interventions in instructor training programs.

As Kristine Newhall argues, more trainings are needed for fitness instructors that focus on feminist approaches and methods. Newhall suggests a more "interdisciplinary" approach to instructor training programs would go toward "engendering a critical consciousness in instructors" (75).[8] Such trainings are needed in most fitness settings in gyms as well as private studios, community centers as well as universities. Better instructor training means providing instructors with feminist tools and concepts and, at the very least, asking instructors to consider feminism as an approach that improves their teaching in a variety of ways. Sometimes instructors' fitness can be unbalanced even as it might comply to the conventional images and meanings of fitness. Because fitness instructors are the glue between programs and participants, Newhall argues that "using instructors as a starting point for challenging fitness industry hegemony allows for the possibility of change in many directions" (75). Initiating this change in the direction of participants is much easier than initiating change in the direction of program coordinators, CEOs, manufacturers, and the industry itself. Support for feminist training might come from academic influence and intervention — particularly where our lives cross these spaces — but also need to be accepted at the local level of fitness — at clubs, gyms, fitness centers, community centers, and other places/spaces for fitness — as well as the industry leaders like Les Mills and Body Training Systems and certification bodies like American Council of Exercise, American Fitness Association of America, and American College of Sports Medicine. In these spaces, feminism exists without being named.

Creating "feminist environment" is a bigger challenge that might include infrastructure and management; however, "feminist environment" can be created in enclaves, in people and places that might be hostile to feminism outside the realm where fitness is happening. Ultimately, an "overall paradigm shift" is the biggest challenge. All throughout this book I am trying to interrupt and re-imagine the current paradigms of "fitness," to create an individual and collective starting point to approach fitness through a feminist lens, toward feminist methods, purposes, tools, and results that can change our body/bodies and our body's/bodies' relationship to the world.

* * *

While feminist fitness is a key to fitness instruction in terms of changing individuals' experiences as well as the industry, feminist fitness principles can certainly be applied to an individual's approach to fitness. Even for those who might find the idea of fitness intimidating, impossible, or uninteresting, there are ways that fitness can be incorporated into their lives through exercise and what are often referred to as "mindfulness" techniques. The fitness enthusiast can also apply ideas of feminist fitness to their workout routine. Recognizing the feeling of meaningful movement, interacting with each other in ways that show respect to ourselves and others, and joining a running community are just a few endeavors toward feminist fitness. But, regardless of individual tools toward feminist fitness, we need better feminist fitness resources.

Searching for Feminist Fitness

Gina Kolata sets out on a "quest for truth about exercise and health" that speaks to the interests of the average American. Despite Kolata's positive relationship with fitness, and her relation of an experience with fitness from the perspective of a female body, she makes no claims toward feminism, and women and/or gender draw no special attention in her quest. This is not unusual in many fitness-oriented stories, studies, or analyses. Despite the comparative wealth of scholarship devoted to women and fitness, and the growing body of feminist inquiries into fitness, we might still wonder how to find feminism "at the gym" or in stacks of magazines and DVDs or in an endless chain of web links. Perhaps we don't even know "feminism" is what we're looking for. Feminist tools and endeavors may be cloaked in classes with trendy names, hidden behind several intimidating doors, or obscured by the reigning adherence to standards of thinness and the "perfect body." Even if we know what we're looking for—a workout that is effective and enjoyable and doesn't reinforce dominant ideas of weight and beauty—it might be hard to find. Many women's resources—magazines, websites, programs—profess to have women's health and maybe even empowerment as part of their agenda. There is an overwhelming amount of fitness-related information ripe for the taking.

Still, there is a lack of helpful information that approaches exercise specifically, and fitness generally, from a feminist perspective. The internet has become a more helpful tool, but the best advice is not necessarily filed under the term "feminist." For instance, Oprah's website provides advice and perspectives that are pro-women, even as they still require a critical eye (like any other pop culture fitness site). In an article from July 2008 in *Oprah Magazine* (and posted on Oprah.com), "Weight Loss: How Women Do the Math," Catherine Price suggests the need for a "personal body image index"—a PBII instead of a BMI. The idea undercuts unrelenting standards and limiting expectations. While a bit flippant in her creative math examples, her advice is helpful toward moving away from narrow standards of the BMI scale. But it also reinforces the need to measure ourselves by *some* standard, even if it is not as strict or harsh as the BMI. She concludes, "When it comes to my own PBII, I still have a way to go.... But recognizing the illogical logic behind my self-image helps me to control it better." Control is still the guiding force, as well as her comparison to other women (older and younger) as a way to feel better about ourselves. She leads us to believe that older women are non-competitive and reinforce youthful qualities, while younger women are insecure and provide liberation. Certainly there is better advice out there?

An interesting example of the rough edge of fitness advice comes from a posting made to Feministing.com by Megan Wade in September of 2009. She explains how she and her mother are looking to start working out and wonders if there are any feminist books that might help them get started. She writes, "So I thought I would turn to the Feministing community for help. Are there fitness or exercise guides out there that you think come from strong feminist perspective? Or ones that aren't explicitly so, but implicitly celebrate women's bodies in their approach? Do you have an exercise guide you especially like to use?" This call is telling since such works are certainly not easy to find, even via the internet and especially among the thousands of choices. But, more interesting are the responses she gets. Only one offers a book example while several offer websites or DVDs, and most agree that books are not the place to look for such advice.

One community member offers: "Dr. Miriam Nelson has written a series of books on the importance of strength training and exercise for women." She provides the link to the book's description on Amazon.com and continues, "I don't specifically remember if it had a feminist slant, but the overall theme was lifelong health rather than losing weight or looking good." Interestingly, this response does not include the full title of the book, *Strong Women Stay Young*, which should offer enough of a clue about the book's approach. This book may be a helpful tool and it certainly boasts powerful results to Dr. Miriam Nelson's program; however, the book description provides a look at this book's agenda: "From the famed research labs of Tufts University, here's a *scientifically proven* strength-training program that *turns back the clock* for women aged 35 and up —*replacing* fat with muscle, *reversing* bone loss, increasing strength and energy, improving balance and flexibility — all in *just* two at-home sessions per week" (my emphasis). Here we find not only the assumption that women need to "turn back the clock" and the authority of science and medicine, but also the promise that it will be "easy." The program and the results are commendable while the package is certainly far from feminist.

Another response, from Jane, is interesting in that it assumes that science is not usually feminist but that it is important knowledge ("yay science!") and it also places value on "kick-your-ass" as a state of desirable fitness. She illuminates the fact that "women's fitness (measured by how much they can lift, how fast they run, how fast they can do a loaded road march, etc)" can improve while body fat percentage might not *substantially change.*" Jane thinks this is "awesomely feminist, and also SCIENCE." Jane's response is providing information related to what Emily's post asked for, and claiming feminist information as well, and yet it is not helpful toward Emily's desires to begin a workout program with her mother. It also reveals the ambivalence surrounding feminist perceptions of fitness, valuing strength above other important benefits. Moreover, it reinforces food, not exercise, as the key to reducing the dreaded enemy — fat. Here, strength and power is portrayed as "feminist."

The most interesting, and potentially helpful, response to Megan's post comes from i_muse. She argues that there is nothing inherently sexist about traditional exercises like walking, jogging, Pilates, or climbing and that there is nothing sexist about a treadmill. She writes, "get up and go is not something you'll find in a book." She then shares the fact that she is a feminist and has years of experience teaching a variety of fitness and, from this experience, the best advice she has to offer is "simply the more you move around the better." While i_muse is right on in this advice, her advice that follows is vague, which is understandable for a comment on a blog. But her tone is not helpful in the least. This post also makes several assumptions like the assumption that motivation is what Megan lacks rather than a lack of knowledge (when she was asking for sources of knowledge). This assumption of a lack of motivation is a pillar in fitness though certainly problems of motivation have multiple layers. Her list of credentials means that "add[ing] some stretching" seems like a rather simple thing to do, and her claim of "the most feminist instruction [she] can offer" from her experience illustrates her authority in a way that seems dismissive. She suggests yoga as an "overall health form" but offers no advice or resources that might help Megan pursue this form. For someone unfamiliar with fitness, figuring out how to stretch, what to stretch, and how long to stretch requires some guidance. Finding the right kind of yoga can feel overwhelming. The biggest letdown of this response, however, is her last line. While demonstrating an anti-consumerist stance that is helpful to avoid the pitfalls of the fitness market monster ("don't spend your money on a book or magazines"), it also offers flippant advice to "go for a walk." Again, this is good advice delivered poorly. Simply adding the idea that walking is an easy way to get started with physical fitness goals and also a great way for Emily and her mom to spend time together would have been a better — and more "feminist"—way to share this fitness knowledge. Here, "not sexist" stands in for "feminist."

If we are searching for feminist fitness, we most often get versions of not sexist, or build strength to gain power, or a woman wrote it so close enough. If we continue looking, we find that some feminist fitness figures share their knowledge, experience, and insights through blogs. Several fabulous blog examples are posted by Fit Feminist ("A blog about random feminist stuff, with a bit of a fitness industry bent."), Fit and Feminist ("Because it takes strong women to smash the patriarchy"), Fat Feminist Fitness Blog, and Feminist Figure Girl. Fit and Feminist provides a number of blogs that feature active women and sound advice with a lean toward athletics. She critiques the ways in which women are portrayed in sports and fitness and provides commentary on her own forays into fitness like trying out a pole dancing class or open water swimming. In her "about" section, Caitlin writes,

> Seeing as though I am about as hardcore a feminist as I am a runner, I can't help but make observations about health, weight, bodies, fitness and sports, particularly as they relate to gender. Rarely a day passes that I don't think about the lack of women in the weight room or consider the harmful effects of the diet industry on the self image of women and girls. So I figured, why not blog about it?

Fit Feminist (Keira), an Australian personal trainer, writes about a number of issues including violence against women, books of interest, politics, and fitness. Her profile describes her as: "I'm a vegan, feminist personal trainer who is into keeping fit, baking, social justice, good books and hot chocolate." Fit Feminist's fitness-related posts include everything from advice like "Quick, effective at-home workout for older women (and the rest of us!)" and critiques like "What's with the Boobs?" Balancing practical and critical advice, this blog provides some feminist fitness insights.

Fat Feminist Fitness Blog provides a much more pronounced feminist agenda. Thealogian writes, "In this blog I hope to track my adventures in fitness, food justice, gardening and body acceptance. I will do so with a critical eye — examining how anti-fat bias, economics, class, sexism, urban (suburban and rural) development deprives us of satisfying movement, and how health is collective and personal." She writes about her own personal goals, offers "vintage beauties" like the cast of Punky Brewster, critiques and comments on pop culture stories like the controversy over Rihanna's "Man Down" video (and Gabrielle Union's related response), and diet-related issues like the problems with Diet Coke Addiction.[9] The critical, practical, and whole-life approach, coupled with an honest voice provides a valuable feminist perspective.

Feminist Figure Girl's site begins to establish an infrastructure for interactive support and advice. It includes blogs, menus and recipes, ask a trainer, guest bloggers, and a glossary. Feminist Figure Girl, whose alter ego is a professor of History of Art, Design, and Visual Culture at the University of Alberta (Lianne McTavish), describes her Feminist Figure Girl work:

> in 2010 [I] decided to combine my identities (scholar/gym rat) to create Feminist Figure Girl, a bodybuilding honey badger. I started this blog when I was training and dieting for my first figure competition, held in June of 2011. I have now written a book inspired by this process, and have submitted it for publication to an academic press. This blog is filled with feminist reflections on food, working out, sexuality, and bodies, and is now collaborative....

Before finishing her book and changing the description, McTavish, notes that she will "document [her] embodied experiences of these activities, but [she] will mostly make fun of [her]self." Her sense of humor about this work is counter to stereotypes about humorless feminists, and is important for disrupting stereotypes about women in both fitness and comedy. She also mentions the pleasure she gains from her fitness activities is equal to that she gains from her academic activities. This site begins to build an online feminist community through Professor McTavish's personal journey. She provides a model for balancing fitness and professional life in tandem with each other. She, and all of these feminist fitness bloggers, model aspects of feminist fitness in online spaces.

One of the best online resources I have found in my searches, I found by accident — Pirkko Markula's blog hosted by Psychologytoday.com, "Fit Femininity: exploring the intersection of culture, gender, and exercise." While rather scholarly in its tone and structure (her "Ph.D." title accompanies her byline), these blogs are shorter and more accessible than academic articles are, and Markula offers a wealth of advice and reflections with a feminist approach. The bio related to the blog explains her qualitative research regarding "women's exercise experiences" and her interests include "the intersections of health, dance, and mindful fitness." Blog topics deal with a variety of issues from common questions that women might have about exercise like what to do when even the modifications for exercise are too difficult, or whether strength training is beneficial, or why we are so afraid of fat. She also reviews and complements work by others in academia or in fitness. For instance, she writes about what other scholars have written about striptease aerobics and standardized exercise classes; she examines the work of a female bodybuilder who offers workout advice for men; and she interviews a friend and fellow academic about his recent Les Mills training experience. She also writes about trends like barefoot running and ultramarathons. Markula's work here is accessible and refreshing; she often considers enjoyment of exercise and offers insights and advice that clarify many of the myths surrounding women and fitness.

For those who are searching for feminist fitness, the most helpful resources come from women who are blogging about their experience, but such resources could certainly be expanded and made more visible and accessible. A forum on Feministing.com offers a potentially productive space for sharing such resources while it also illustrates that regardless of the format, few overtly feminist resources exist. "Feminist Fitness" has appeared on Tumblr, providing an overt focus on "all shapes and sizes" and "body-positive fitness and diet tips" and an invitation to contribute to the site. Academic knowledge outside the "hard" sciences is still in the process of radiating through the world of fitness (rather than trickling down), making connections and challenging assumptions. Creating more resources, more spaces to search for and access such resources, and more demand for feminist approaches to fitness are some of the ways that we can contribute to knowledge production and sharing of that knowledge, within and beyond feminist circles. While *Women and Fitness in American Culture* does not include sample workouts, diet plans, or step-by-step instructions, it does aim to be a resource — applied, adapted, extended, and internalized as necessary.

Sketches: Transformative Innovators: Making Belly Dance Work Out

As dance aerobics have developed, a variety of dance forms have influenced, and been adapted by, aerobics and have created a variety of fitness dance forms and formats. Belly Dance fitness forms range across a spectrum of productions, levels of effectiveness, and talent of instructors. Some have more of a fitness focus; others more dance focus. Such forms are most accessible via DVD or online video such as "SharQuí: The Bellydance Workout," created by Oreet or "Bellydance: Fitness for Weight Loss" featuring Ranía. In some places, these belly dance fitness forms are available at fitness studios, like Hipline in northern California.

When a co-worker loaned me a SharQuí DVD, I had no idea of the power and magic I would experience. Oreet's DVD is truly the best fitness DVD I have seen — the most real, the most comfortable, the most organic. Oreet encourages her participants in the low-budget studio with her and those who are watching this experience on DVD. She provides instruction that is peppered with reminders of beauty. Oreet exudes confidence and inspiration. This fitness brand does not fall into the trap of American fitness ideals as does that featuring Ranía. While Ranía's DVDs promise weight loss, Oreet's promise is "the most body-loving and soul-stimulating elements from the art form of belly dance" combined with "the burn that an aerobic workout can offer." Its goal is not "increasing metabolism" but helping us to "feel good on the inside and out." Her DVD has this impact as the women look real and are diverse (in size, shape, and color), the movements are performed in a way that is easy to follow, and Oreet's encouragement feels genuine rather than scripted. After the warm-up and routine, the DVD concludes with an "improv" section where the four women in the workout video and Oreet dance together in a way that highlights the roots of belly dance as a social and cultural art shared by groups and communities of women. One dancer is centered while the others cheer her on and each woman has an opportunity to be both center and periphery.

Oreet's bio on the original DVD relates the story that Oreet brought her love and talent for dance to New York's fitness clubs. When she felt that something was missing, she went back "to her [Middle East] roots" as she combined fitness and dance with the "body-loving art form of belly dance." She found that the workouts in fitness classes may have worked the body but they left an "unsatisfied sense of well-being." Essentially, Oreet has put a mind/body bandage on aerobics. She found a way to create a sense of well-being through dance in her classes and she encapsulated this message through her DVD version of this "bellydance workout." She "continues to expose women to Shar-Quí's philosophy and methods," offering master classes and creating more DVDs like the 2009 level one version of SharQuí.

In the original DVD, Oreet uses the other women to demonstrate technique, she interacts with them and each woman is part of the whole picture and an individual dancer. On the 2009 DVD, Oreet has two dancers behind her (like many typical fitness DVDs) and she is the center and the only voice as she cues the movements. After the cool-down segment of the DVD, a performance section of the DVD features Oreet, reinforcing belly dance as a performance art and showcasing the art of movement that can be enhanced through the SharQuí fitness workout. It does not highlight the "perfect body" but the beauty of movement, art, and technique. Unlike the original DVD, this focus on performance also means a focus on the individual art of belly dance rather than the community tradition, a feature that speaks to the iconic, personality-driven nature of the fitness industry rather than the communal nature of dance and fitness. Regardless, Oreet's DVD is a whole package that innovates upon a fitness form so that it can offer much more — a means toward transformation.

Finding Oreet had me searching for other belly dance fitness examples. I came across Hipline, a belly dance fitness system and studio created by sisters, Samar and Gabriela Nassar, from Oakland, California. What they had created was impressive, but when I came back to the site a couple years later, Hipline had grown. Hipline Dance Fitness — the site and the business — is more developed and the signature class, Shimmy Pop had expanded into other forms like Shimmy Pop Toning and Shimmy Flow, an Arabic dance class. Hipline also has two studios, Rockridge, in Berkeley, and Lakeshore, in Oakland. Hipline includes two-hour workshops along with their regular one-hour classes. They also offer a Dance Jungle Playroom for children several times a week. They've put together a Hipline Flash mob to invade the Grand Lakes Farmer's market. And when a new instructor joins the studio, they feature and promote her first class as a free event. These kinds of events help to build community and provide ways to get involved in movement outside of studio classes.

The website and newsletter, as well as the Vimeo channel also help to strengthen the Hipline community. In a 2012, Reader's Poll for the *East Bay Express*, Hipline was name the "Most Subversive Exercise Routine." As Hipline choreographer, Heather, notes, "due to our unique approach to fitness (yay!)." This unique approach comes from a team of sixteen choreographers/instructors, a diverse group of women who bring their own flavor and personality to the Shimmy Pop style. The very inviting and friendly website provides information about choreographers and classes, including important updates and short sample videos. In one August 2012 update, Hipline reminds participants how much work it is to balance 50 classes and making sure instructors/choreographers are "being well taken care of so they can give their best performances."

In this update, they remind Hipliners to "be like water" as classes change and subs are needed to fill in. They conclude the update with a YouTube link to Bruce Lee speaking his philosophy on water, "be formless, shapeless, like water ... you put water into a bottle, it becomes the bottle ... water can flow or it can crash. Be water, my friend." These sentiments offer important messages about Hipline. First, they care about their instructors and want to remind participants to care about them as well. Sometimes we get so locked into the love of our favorite fitness class that we forget that instructors should also listen to their bodies and be healthy. In fact, referring to their instructors as choreographers shows a degree of respect for the talent it takes to put together a cardio dance class. And the more we are all "like water" not only can we move better in the studio, but we can move better through life. These are powerful messages to couple with fitness.

But Hipline provides many powerful messages, as choreographer, Heather, explains, "what we do goes way beyond exercise. Hipline is a Movement. It is a community of phenomenal women with whom we get to learn amazing life lessons from this art form we lovingly call Shimmy Pop." She shares her "top ten" lessons in an August 2012 post including: "love your body, let go of perfection, connect, take up space, move through challenges, and breathe." These lessons speak to a feminist fitness approach, even though Heather does not describe it as such. At the end of her list she concludes: "In each class and in every day, find ways to be authentically yourself: to be brave, to get lost, to flirt, to have some 'therapeutic moments,' to show your sassy attitude, to toot your own horn, to be however you need it to be in the most beautiful, bold and courageous ways. *Allow dance to be a platform to change your life.*" (She shares some of this wisdom on her own website, "Create Your Own Beautiful," making Heather a fitness innovator in her own right.) She recognizes that dance can be a "platform" for transformation and Hipline certainly works to give their community such tools.

The videos on the website introduce the "Hipspiration" of the month as well as short combinations. Viewers can not only get a taste of the class and the instructor's style, they can also learn skills that are applicable in the classes. In each video the choreographer describes the moves, performs them to music, and invites the viewer to join her at Hipline. The July 2012 Hipspiration was inspired by Lady Gaga's "Born This Way." Co-founder, Samar, introduces an undulation combo and tells viewers, "... here at Hipline we celebrate our differences. Everybody moves different ... definitely put your own flavor on top of it because that's how we do it here ... [laughs]." In an interview in the online Newsletter for Hipline, new Arabic Dance (Shimmy Flow) teacher, Rebecca, describes what she loves about Hipline: "What I love about Hipline is that it really encourages you to be your own woman. Samar and Gabriela have made a space where you can appreciate yourself and each other. My favorite aspect of the studio is that Hipline has created a really positive environment where women can express themselves in dance." When I visit the website and watch the videos, Northern California seems so achingly far away. Not only have these women built a business, they have built a space where women can express themselves freely and in a fun and empowering way.

My Generation and Beyond

The relationship that I have with fitness, the way I feel about going to the gym, has been built upon a feminist foundation established by my mother and her generation. We have been allowed to do things with our bodies that were frowned upon or outright prohibited for past generations. We have been encouraged in participation even as we have been discouraged by unequal playing fields, literally and figuratively. We have been able to see the possibilities in fitness. We have felt the effects of activity and movement from youth and we have been encouraged to express ourselves. We have a different relationship to these ideas and less cultural baggage to weigh us down. And yet, fitness is largely relegated to individual pursuits, government mandates, and community initiatives.

Of course, not all members of my generation feel the same way and a variety of circumstances will alter one's points of reference regarding fitness. Along those lines of class, race, and gender, our experiences with, and opportunities for, fitness or sports often mirror society's patterns and hierarchies, even as these experiences are varied. Regardless of these dividers, members of my fitness generation are wedded to women outside of our generation and generational lines blur when we are all sweating and moving together. In the fitness classes that I teach and take at the YMCA, the ages vary from 14 (the minimum age for most group exercise classes) to the mid–70s. Sometimes younger girls take my classes, and many YMCAs also include youth fitness programs and programs like Silver Sneakers, the most widely available fitness program for older adults in the U.S. Generations work out together.

* * *

I was born on the edge of generations — far behind the first Generation Xers, those who set the stage and defined a generation as much as their generation was named and shaped by the Baby Boomers. In my introductory sociology class my first year of college (in 1994) we learned about "Generation X" (with birth dates from the mid 1960s through the late 70s) and read and watched some of the seminal works of this generation like Douglas Rushkoff's *The Gen X Reader* and the film *Reality Bites*. Rushkoff explains in his introduction to *The GenX Reader*: "Generation X means a lot of things to a lot of people. We are a culture, a demographic, an outlook, a style, an economy, a scene, a political ideology, an aesthetic, an age, a decade, and a literature" (3). He explains that this book is the first time that Generation X has been able to speak for itself since "it has always been explained to the public by the people who fear and detest us most" (4). Despite the fact that I didn't really identify with the public image or self-definition of Generation X, Rushkoff's message resonated with me. I had not (yet) "dropped out of American culture as traditionally defined" but I did see my generation as "a testament to American ingenuity, optimism, instinct, and brilliance" (4).

I identified with some of the same cultural markers of this generation like *Star Wars*, *The Brady Bunch* (in reruns), and *The Simpsons*. There were also things I did not share with those GenXers, mainly the "slacker" mentality, but also some key events and trends that I was too young to experience or understand. Much later I learned that the Generation X group identity is splintered as both the Hip Hop Generation and the generation of Third Wave Feminists claim the same span of birth dates. All three are identities, rooted in cultures — popular and local. I identify with cultural markers from these generational conceptualizations as well, like Run DMC and Madonna, respectively. But because of my age, my class, and my somewhat sheltered upbringing, I missed out on important cultural markers like the career and death of Tupac and the rise of the Riot Grrrls.[10] Simultaneously, my generation is shaped by these divisive pictures of race and gender identification even as it shares some common cultural texts and events, belief systems and assumptions. These are issues that my generation has had to work out, and we are a conflicted generation.

* * *

The first glimpse that I got of academic ideas about fitness was expressed by Third Wave feminist, Alisa L. Valdés, in "Ruminations of a Feminist Fitness Instructor" in *Listen Up: Voices from the Next Feminist Generation.*[11] If she was a part of my generation, and technically she was, our experiences in fitness were separated by class, ethnicity, location, personal/career aspirations, and approach/meaning of fitness in our lives. While she experienced fitness as an oppressive patriarchal regime, I experienced it as powerful and empowering, as a tool and a means to make people — and myself— feel better. But the problems with Valdés's views of fitness also illustrate some of the fissures in my generation, particularly along the lines of the personal/political.

Valdés begins her article with the premise that the title of "feminist aerobics instructor" is absurd. "It's like being a fascist poet. People think you can't" (25). The problem with being a fitness instructor, she argues, is that she "watched as [her] life-long dream of being a professional feminist writer slipped through [her] fingers and back into [her] spandex and sneakers, all because [she] needed to pay for a roof over [her] head and the food in [her] stomach" (28–9). She could not find balance between dreams of being a feminist writer and the economic realities that drove her to have to be a "*professional* instructor" (27; original emphasis). But she wasn't simply a fitness instructor, she was a fitness *celebrity*: "teaching at the city's top clubs"; training fitness instructors for AFAA; entering an aerobics competition in which she and her male partner "bounced [their] way" to second place; heading an aerobics program; and presenting a master class at the Boston MetroSports

Fitness Expo (27). She almost brags, "people in the industry knew my name" (27).[12]

As she developed this professional fitness life, she also searched feminist theory for some meaning to what she was doing. She cites the work of Iris Marion Young, and her "hero" Robin Morgan, who argue the importance of the body in relation to the intellect. Valdés writes:

> I think that maybe this is why I taught, as well: to dance, to connect with my body in a tangible way so that I could better connect with my intellect and assist others in doing the same. The process of strengthening the body could also strengthen women's ability to achieve our goals. Never mind that those goals — to achieve that flat tummy, to fit into that tiny wedding dress, to lose ten pounds before going to Club Med to find Mr. Right — do not exactly subvert the patriarchy. Creating a psychological space where women could move, really move, was the thrill [30].

Even as she recognizes empowerment, Valdés cites these limiting goals which are, of course, extensions of mainstream, patriarchal expectations of women's fit bodies that women have internalized. (The same espoused by Cooper and LL Cool J.) And, overall, Valdés's ultimate conclusion that "none of us, instructors or members, will ever reach our real goals playing by the rules of that industry" (32), is absolutely correct. The problems, as she illustrates, are structured not only into the fitness industry, but the larger culture as well. She could pay back her student loans, but she felt a "gnawing ache of betrayal" (28). Because these are structural problems, the industry that Valdés enters upon finishing graduate school and becoming a writer is ruled by the same contradictions as the fitness industry. Valdés, in part, convinced me of the legitimacy of feminist fitness even as she denounced its possibilities.

In the 20 plus years since the publication of this article, Valdes's life has taken many turns and she has, in fact, become a successful writer, winning awards and recognition. Until 2001, she wrote for newspapers and magazines including *The Boston Globe* (the job that concludes her ruminations), *The Los Angeles Times*, and *Glamour* and *Redbook*. And Valdes has found great success through her writing, categorized as "Chick Lit." Her first book, *Dirty Girls Social Club*, sparked a publisher's bidding war and placed her on the *NY Times* bestseller's list for 21 weeks. She has also published other books in this series, five other novels, some teen fiction, and a "novelita," an on-line erotic e-book that's a "hot, sexy romance series." She continues to write blogs, romance novels, and erotica as well as other related projects.[13]

In late 2012, besides her piece in *Listen Up!*, Valdes's career in fitness was mostly invisible and she had a new book due to be released in early 2013, a memoir that was being heavily promoted. No mention of "Ruminations," or her career in fitness, was made in her bio on her author's page or in a Wikipedia entry about her. It was not even mocked in the "Uncyclopedia" entry that lambasts her for her political views and career choices. Perhaps this fitness past no longer seemed relevant to her new life as a lucrative writer. She was famous not for "hopping around in leotards" (27) but for other more "serious" pursuits. It's what she always wanted. But Valdes's feminism disappeared as well.

In her 2013 memoir titled *The Feminist and the Cowboy: An Unlikely Love Story* we find that not only is Valdes no longer a feminist, but she is anti-feminism. In her blog titled, "Learning to Submit: Questioning Extreme Feminism's Impact on Romance, Love, and Relationships," she explains that she is "a former feminist who has penned a memoir about how feminism stole my womanhood (and the super-charged romance with the traditional cowboy who helped me find it)." In some ways, Valdes's transformation makes sense. In "Ruminations" she is contradicted, conflicted, guilty, angry, and self-righteous, and despite her claims of feminism, she demeans other women who choose to be cheerleaders or women who choose to have careers in fitness rather than more "serious" pursuits like writing. At the forefront of third wave feminists and my generation, "despite her professional success" she found herself, as the book description (for the original title) *Learning to Submit* describes, "forty-two [years old,] a single mom and a serial dater of inadequate men in tweed jackets—until she met the Cowboy." Clearly, something happened between the end of her professional fitness career and her apparently dissatisfying role as a mother and a successful writer to make her ripe for "a conservative rancher, [who] held the traditional views on gender roles that Valdes was raised to reject." Unfortunately, feminism was the scapegoat. And unfortunately, Valdes's story continues to suffer from contradictions connected to feminist fitness.

After the publication of her memoir, Valdes admitted to Salon.com that she was physically, sexually, and emotionally abused by "the cowboy." In an article on thefrisky.com, "On Alisa Valdes' Conflict With Feminism, Her Cowboy & Domestic Abuse," Jessica Wakeman relates Valdes' "sordid tale" which includes quotes from a blog Valdes posted on January 9, 2013 that was later removed. As Wakeman argues, there are several problems with the ways in which Valdes presents her story. Most glaringly, "*The Feminist and the Cowboy* and all Valdes's ensuing blog posts about the relationship read, somewhat sadly, like massive self-justification for being in an abusive relationship." But what concerns me most (and Wakeman too[14]) is that there are many ways that Valdes could have told the real story behind her relationship with the cowboy (and she has mentioned writing a sequel), and yet the story that is being told (and has been told before, and will continue being told) is the one encapsulated by the book description, found widely on Amazon.com and other sites: "The Feminist and the Cowboy will delight ... many readers ... not to mention every woman who dreams of being swept away by a rugged cowboy." Here is where the danger lies.

Valdes admits, in her Buena Vida Blog bio (updated in 2013), that she has "made a lot of mistakes, and learned from them." She has "finally found peace, happiness and a very good life." She shares this life and this story with her readers and here her fitness work has a renewed (though minimal) presence. She has also, apparently, found a type of feminism that works for her: "she maintains her stance as a 'difference feminism' (men and women have separate but equal value and worth)," as Kat Stoeffel observes. And as several articles observe, Valdes has found validation with a new boyfriend. After quoting the Salon.com article where Valdes shared her story of abuse, Wakeman writes "*You read that right: her new boyfriend wrote a thank you note to her abusive, rapist ex-boyfriend thanking him for 'taming' her.*" Maybe Valdes is still working it out. In an April 2, 2013 blog post, "How the Body Reminds the Spirit What Matters," she admits that *The Cowboy and the Feminist* was a "naive and somewhat regrettable memoir." She also talks about her "chronic overachiever" personality and her recently-recognized inability to do it all (which has been an important feminist issue for quite some time). She writes, "I'm not going to let that one book ruin my dreams, or destroy my spirit. I'm going to pick up, and keep writing, because that's what I do best. Writing is why I'm here." She still teaches group fitness (Zumba), which she mentions in this post as well, and intends to do so, she notes, until she can't walk anymore. I feel the same way. Our stories diverge and converge.

* * *

Certainly, my fitness experience was impacted not only by class, race, gender, time, and location, but also by the generation that came before me, a generation that represents itself through the image of Jane Fonda and the rise of dance aerobics programs like Jazzercise, created by Judi Sheppard Missett in 1969, and aerobic dance, created by Jacki Sorensen as she took Cooper's *Aerobics* ideas and put them to music. In the 1980s, Gin Miller created step aerobics after using a step in a rehabilitation program after injuring herself through high-impact aerobics. And in 1992, Mary Swanson created Silver Sneakers, an exercise program for aging adults. All of these women, and more, have set standards for group fitness and aerobics classes.

In her introduction to *My Life at the Gym*, Jo Malin describes returning to/discovering the gym later in life. This was the case for my mother and for many of my participants. For many women, the gym beckons only as they discover that their bodies are aging. Some may have had intermittent experiences, as Myrl Coulter explains in "Gym Interrupted": "after high school, my gym experiences would be interrupted for several years as I got down to the business of finding a husband, and a job to keep me occupied while I did so, activities my family and countless others expected of young women newly graduated from high school in 1968" (103). Some women only find the time to go to the gym when their children have grown and they have more time to devote to themselves. Many of the stories told in *My Life at the Gym* come from this set of experiences, from a generation of women who have had to give themselves permission to care about their health and wellness rather than just their appearance. This is the generation that made that space open for my generation.

I love *My Life at the Gym*; and, yet, when I read it I cannot help but feel like the voice of my generation is only marginally included. Nowhere is this more evident than in Jacqueline Brady's chapter, "Beyond the Lone Images of the Superhuman Strongwoman and Well-Built Bombshell toward a New Communal Vision of Muscular Women." Without citing a single "third-wave" feminist text or voice, Brady discounts and diminishes "these feminists" who "focus on the freedom of self expression," assume revolutionary transformation, and overlook the normalizing practices, conformist aspects, and disciplining aspects of muscular women. (87)

But exclusion and minimalization of Third Wave Feminism makes sense. Fitness trends are dominated by people who have had time to practice and train, to develop systems, and to understand the body (generally and specifically) and the industry. And third-wave feminists have reaped the benefits of these developments. My generation is familiar with these trends, with the rise of mixer music and Reebok's Step Aerobics. We pack the Zumba classes and yoga studios (along with our mothers and daughters). We're committed to a running regimen. We enjoy outdoor activities. We live for CrossFit or P90X. We find empowerment through a variety of activities and, yet, we're beginning to approach that time in our lives when suddenly the gym becomes an obligation and/or a necessity ... or something to be avoided at all costs. Thus, *IDEA Fitness Journal* also found it an opportune time in July/August of 2011, to include an article about my generation: "Generation X: From Slackers to Stars, the Future of Fitness" by Amanda Vogel.

In addition to "workplace fun," Gen X also has a "preference for work-life balance" (34). According to the author's own experiences with "a family of [her] own and a full-time career," for many Gen Xers, "priorities have shifted" (32). Even as these priorities shift for some of us, we continue to incorporate fitness into our lives in ways that we can make it fit. And it turns out that the cynicism that Generation X has been criticized for is "a strength when evaluating trends and fads" (33). It is also a strength in terms of seeing past the sometimes narrow strictures of science. When we design routines or programs, we don't simply listen to the dictates of the experts, we also apply practical knowledge that comes from application of fitness techniques and principles. One of the positive impacts of this orientation to fitness is that "'you're seeing more group exercise classes where everyone is thankfully encouraged to move at a speed appropriate to them'" (33).

All of these thoughts about Generation X are geared toward how to think about the role of this generation in the fitness industry—what kind of programming do Gen Xers want and need and what kind of programming can Gen Xers provide. Vogel sees the potential of Generation X as a bridge between the Baby Boomers and the Millennials. We have taught to "'both sides of [our] generation'" one of Vogel's sources notes, and so we can connect to the generations before ours and after ours; we are both "mature" and "hip." We are proficient in the fitness forms familiar to our parents' generation and we are innovating the fitness forms that connect to our kids. Further, Gen Xers might train the next generation in the fading "art of presentation," (33) Vogel argues. One of her sources notes that today's workouts "'lack the luster'" needed in previous programs. What this seems to be referring to is not the performance style, but the mode of training, the rise of manufactured fitness. Already, the way I learned to teach fitness is referred to as "old school." Creating combos and routines (choreography), innovating on old fitness forms and creating new ones, is becoming, more and more, the work of the few. Thus, our role is to train the next generation in the art of creating choreography and routines and delivering those routines in fun, safe, and accessible ways. These are the fading arts—performance is everywhere.

But Vogel also notes that the Millennial generation "does not appreciate the 'exercise for the sake of exercise' mindset that defined the onset of the fitness movement for Gen Xers" (36). Exercise disguised as gaming or toward a particular purpose, like a 5K, Vogel argues, is the way to reach this next generation. Perhaps the natural progression of manufactured fitness is embodied by the Wii Fit, a fitness video game. The programming includes yoga, strength training, aerobics, and balance games. The system is interactive but *interaction* is not synonymous with *engagement*. As Jaana Parviainen argues, "The user of interactive technologies such as computer games allows the machine to be active on the user's behalf" (53). Interestingly, via use of the balance board, center of balance is a key component of the Wii Fit workouts. Center of Balance is monitored throughout the game and points are deducted if a player fails to maintain a certain threshold. Considering the marginalization of balance in most fitness programs, this is an interesting (and perhaps promising) aspect of the Wii Fit. There is movement happening and body awareness is a part of the experience.

As video game play increases and physical education budgets are cut, there are fewer formalized opportunities for young people to learn about and engage with fitness, especially in foundational ways and in forms beyond traditional sports and games approaches. Tara Brabazon examines one particular example: Cabell Midland High School. At this high school, students take a foundational course in physical education and then can choose from a number of electives in a variety of fitness forms. Brabazon mentions how a men's fitness magazine (*Muscle and Fitness*, September 1998) critiques this school program, in part lamenting that the "'moderate exercise'" that is being promoted is not going to produce good enough health and strength benefits, instead, the author argues, "playing hard is the answer'" (72). This is emblematic of the dominant masculine approach to ideas of fitness, and, as Brabazon corrects this view: "Actually, playing hard after a period of inactivity is the wrong answer. Fitness is built incrementally" (72).

In "Obesity, Body Pedagogies and Young Women's Engagement with Exercise" by Emma Rich, John Evans and Laura De Pian, the authors find that "the girls' engagement with exercise was significantly shaped by the cultural pressures toward an instrumental relationship with exercise instead of experiencing the joy of movement" (155). Thus, the messages that they are getting about exercise mirror other cultural messages and discourage the many benefits of exercise that cannot be easily measured or observed. Movement is measured for its specific results: burning calories, losing weight, building strength, improving flexibility. As with older women, weight or "fat" is of primary concern.

A November 2012 headline proclaimed that "toned teens" of today are trying to build muscle. Reporting the results of a new study that surveyed teens at 20 urban middle and high schools, author Linda Carroll argues that "All those glossy magazine ads showing men — and women — with bulging muscles may be having a big impact on America's youth." The "90 percent of boys and 80 percent of girls [who] said they were exercising to become more buff," is a serious concern, Carroll argues, because they are turning to diets and supplements that are dangerous for kids' bodies and development. Because these survey results are from the St. Paul/Minneapolis area, they can hardly be said to be representative of the whole of teens across America; however, regardless of the sample limitations, the results are worthy of consideration. But can we really assume that the image of toned women "certainly signals a change in what American teens see as the ideal female body"?

There are some girls who are attempting to make a difference not only in their own lives, but also in the lives of other teens and pre-teens. Jessy Lipke, a young Canadian, is the face and inspiration of the "Power Girl Fitness Revolution," which she founded (with the help and support of her parents) at ten years of age. Her Power Girl Fitness website (powergirlfitness.com) shares her message and hope for fitness: the vision, "Better Choices Mean a Better Body and a Better Life!"; and the mantra, "Power, Passion and Performance." The story told on her website is that Jessy noticed that other kids were not making the same kind of choices regarding what they eat and what they do to stay active (watch TV and play video games); "her friends at school and in the 'dance world' struggl[ed] with their weight issues and resultant poor self-images." Jessy noticed that they were being raised differently than she was. In her intro video she notes that "more kids than ever before already have bad habits by the age of eight" and are making "bad lifestyle choices" and "developing adult diseases." She continues, "the sad reality is that we are part of the first generation of kids in history who will not outlive our parents unless we make major lifestyle changes." This is all true enough, and coming from the mouth of another kid, this advice might be easier to swallow. But, the assumption here that "weight issues and resultant poor self-images" are caused by the way they are raised is a contradiction. Personal responsibility for kids and teens is transferred to parents. In fact, Jessy's concern is for kids all around the world; however, the "sad realities" of this generation are isolated and glossed over.

The introduction to Jessy further explains that:

> while studying the "experts," she noticed that there was no program to allow girls to have community and connection with other girls in the fitness world. It seemed as though, to get fit, you had to wait until you were an adult to be coached by an adult, or pretend that you were one already and follow along with an adult class, hoping not to injure yourself in the process.

The exercise and nutrition programs that Jessy teaches and promotes, as "your friend and coach" are "doctor designed fun and effective fitness." The programs are "taught for girls, by girls" but they are designed by her parents — her father, a chiropractor and personal trainer, and her mother, a nutritionist. And certainly the things Jessy says and the descriptions on the website have a heavy parental hand. Jessy's appearance is also rather adult — decked out in mid-drifts and hoop earrings — and she and her friends are very skinny.[15] The site and products are still in process and while there are a lot of fitness buzz words like a promise to share all her parents' "secrets" and offer "new and exciting" workouts every month, there is also some sound advice. Not surprisingly, the same language that pervades the adult world — that of personal responsibility — is rampant here. While Jessy credits her parents for her good choices and the knowledge she is sharing, there is no mention of the parental influence on the children who are making bad decisions. It's implied, but parents are let off the hook, just as culture is let off the hook, and the kids then become responsible for their own "lifestyle choices." A responsible choice is, apparently, to purchase Power Girl Fitness workouts and join the community.

Power Girl Fitness is certainly a far cry from the "Get In Shape Girl" toys of my youth and certainly takes advantage of the technological tools at the disposal of many young girls, even if such access might be limited to *some* girls "all over the world." The site is, however, far more inviting than girlshealth.gov which offers an array of advice related to health and fitness in a voice that is clearly coming from an adult. Girls' voices are important and if we want girls to embrace fitness, we should certainly listen and find ways in which movement can speak to girls in their own language(s). The next generation needs guidance to balance the demands of manufactured fitness and the potential for transformation. My generation can model and animate feminist fitness to young people.

The next generation is probably served best by more grassroots programs that serve girls locally. Fitness-based programs for youth are important to develop healthy ideas of fitness and healthy relationships with one's body. Sports camps that specialize in hockey or cheer or soccer are not the same as a focus on fitness. As we grow fitness programs, we empower the next generation to approach fitness not simply from their couches or from the vantage of competitive physical activities. Moreover, because "exercise and physical activity practices associated with new health imperatives tend to homogenize young people's diverse interests, needs and opportunities across ethnicity, class, age, culture and ability" (Rich, et al.) we need to be sure to address such differences by developing and funding local fitness programs that meet youth where they are, without applying cookie-cutter models. We want to engender a love of fitness, not stunt its growth.

Belly Dance as Tool and Springboard

"Amid the jungle of confusing women's images, belly dancing can help women in the search for their own identity, as women and as human beings."

"To perform belly dancing, it does not matter whether a woman is young or old, fat or thin, socially integrated or marginal. Belly dancing is not a competition — competing is not part of its nature. This dance form is more than just a dance. Only a woman's life experience and sensuality can lend it both meaning and true depth."
— Rosina-Fawzia Al-Rawi, *Grandmother's Secrets* (viii, 63)

Belly dancing is a form of dance that has been performed by women from ancient times into the present, all around the world, particularly in the Middle East. It is inherently feminist despite its "sexy" reputation in Western popular culture. When I subbed a children's dance class and introduced some basic belly dance movements, one parent lectured me after class about how she didn't want her daughter to learn to move her hips "that way." Another parent refused to let her special needs daughter return the next week despite the obvious benefits the girl found. She was focused, graceful, and calm. Her eyes cried to me as her mom pulled her away by the arm. The mothers' cultural baggage made them interpret the movements differently from the way the children experienced these movements.

In my Introduction to Women's Studies class we spend a semester getting acquainted with feminism, understanding the workings of power, critiquing social constructions and media representations, and then we learn about belly dancing. Teaching about belly dancing in women's studies classes brings together a variety of topics that we discuss throughout class including: body image and beauty, global feminisms, feminist spirituality, mother/daughter relationships, cross-cultural connections and difference, girls' studies, pop feminism, and cultural expressions, representations, and negotiations. Students read *Grandmother's Secrets* as well as bell hooks chapters about love and spirituality from *Feminism Is for Everybody*. We discuss love and spirituality as well as dancing through discussion and movement. We critique pop culture examples from video clip examples — from more traditional styles of belly dancing, to Hilary Duff on *So You Think You Can Dance*, to a male belly dancer, to a pregnant woman's celebration of her body through belly dance. After critiquing mainstream standards of beauty, students are able to recognize and appreciate a different view of beauty — an embodied beauty.

Critiquing belly dancing in mainstream media creates opportunities to talk about cultural appropriation and sexualization of women in popular culture. It also leads to discussions about body image and cultural expectations and the ways in which women challenge limiting representations. My first semester, when we were reviewing video clips of belly dancing, one student remarked about the size of the women. *They're all skinny.* She was right. In my other two sections of the same class we had critiqued body representations but we had not considered size. The thin bodies of these dancers was sending an unrealistic image, as media (the internet) tends to do. Since then I have incorporated different clips, including pregnant women, and we always discuss the belly's role in body image and popular culture.

Learning about belly dancing forces students to confront many of their preconceived stereotypes about women from the Middle East being victims of oppression. After reading "Global Women's Studies: An Essay in Three Life-Stories" by Rita S. Kranidis, from *An Interdisciplinary Introduction to Women's Studies*, students read Rosina's childhood stories, spent among women and shaped by dance. Their preconceived notions of "women from other countries," as students often generalize, or Middle Eastern women, in this case specifically, are shattered. The ideas of abused and dominated women are disrupted by the empowered community of women who raise Rosina-Fawzia. This compassion helps them to see both cultural specificity and cultural difference as well as cross-cultural connections and shared understandings. This is one of Al-Rawi's hopes about her book, and about belly dancing more generally, she writes, "by experiencing unfamiliar movements, a woman can allow her body to break through cultural norms" (viii). In WST 101, Al-Rawi's book provides this opportunity and then an opportunity to practice "unfamiliar movements." Whether as a result of knowledge or dance, students are moved. Belly dancing in a fitness setting is empowering in ways that belly dancing in the academic classroom will never be. And yet, ideas from the academic realm can enhance the practice of conscious movement in fitness spaces.

Students, often reluctantly, participate in a "head-to-toe" introduction to belly dancing to conclude our discussion. We stand up and we move. This penultimate class is often students' favorite, and students who were not excited about the topic previously often change their minds or at least learn something new. Some don't really try to experience this kinesthetic pedagogy while most smile and giggle and create a new relationship with their body.[16] Perhaps they are not ready for this "physical awareness" that Al-Rawi argues can also spur psychological awareness. Some, not enough, students pursue belly dancing after taking WST 101 and report the pleasure and empowerment they find in this movement. But even when students don't pursue the practice, they find relevance, make connections, and develop respect for other cultural practices. One student made connections to her indigenous/Penobscot traditions, finding similarities in movements and meanings. Another shared her longing to grow up in a culture and household that celebrated dance and shared a story about how her father would conflate dancing with "whoring around." She and her mother, aunts, and their friends celebrated her 21st birthday and her mother's divorce with a night of dancing. One of the few men brave enough to take my WST 101 class, and brave enough to join us for belly dancing, noted the spiritual aspects of belly dancing and compared these to the benefits he finds from walking. He concludes that there is power and connection and a potential for love in belly dancing similar to the benefits he finds through other gender-neutral movements like walking.

* * *

We never know where our tools might come from and the best fitness instructors draw inspiration from trying new physical activities. Belly dancing is something that I was never really exposed to throughout my life and never had an opportunity to see, much less to experience. I never really considered pursuing something like belly dancing — something so much freer, something so different from group fitness. And yet, when I had the opportunity to take some classes when I was in Minnesota for a year, I ventured out of my comfort zone and joined a gymnasium full of women who were all, for the most part, younger and thinner and some more coordinated. But I did not let that intimidate me as I would have in the past. The crowd slowly dwindled as the session wound down, and I was surprised at how much I learned and how much I grew from that belly dancing class. First I learned about belly dance through movement and then through theory.

Immediately I fell in love with the movements of belly dancing. The moves were a new challenge. I had to work hard; I had to push my body to move in ways that I had not moved before. I had to train my body out of the little, linear box that fitness had put me in. And in doing this, belly dancing also opened up a new perspective on fitness. I began to see the ways in which the movements from belly dancing could be taught in a cardio format. I practiced the belly dancing moves that I learned in class in front of a narrow mirror in my small, mostly empty apartment. I practiced to Hip Hop music, the kind of music I most enjoy and the kind of music with the most predominant beat to follow. I would recreate the movements from memory, take home what I had learned in class.

Some kernels of cardio belly dance routines were born, but I had neither the time nor the opportunity to develop them until later. There was a learning curve — choosing the right song, creating the best movements, recognizing the song's structure, memorizing the parts and matching choreography to the music, cuing it all effectively ... and then putting together enough songs to make a whole class. This experience was similar to when I began to learn how to teach fitness classes. I would choreograph routines to songs from my small collection of music (until mixer music was introduced to me). I had to dust off and embellish these skills for cardio belly dancing; I was creating a specific routine for a specific song and I would mold the movements according to my experience of the music. Each song/routine was an organic process of discovering belly dance movement. I found that what I really loved about fitness was this experience of creating — and belly dancing, in its innovative qualities, is the perfect form to use to create.

Bringing this fitness form into the academic classroom is a space where the toolbox overlaps and where feminist fitness takes root.

* * *

One of the ways in which I highlight the feminist aspects of belly dancing is to infuse some belly dance wisdom into group fitness classes that are really focused on skills and practice or cardiovascular endurance. For instance, when doing shoulder exercises I discuss how moods are revealed by our shoulders "carrying worries on your shoulders" (100). Women carry many responsibilities and recognizing this helps us to make connections between our daily lives and the movements we are doing. As we learn to move our shoulders more freely we can begin to shrug off our worries more easily as well. And our worries manifest in many different parts of our bodies. With belly dancing's focus on isolations we can examine each part of our body separately. "Neck tensions," Al-Fawzi reminds us, "usually arise from a fear of failing, of making mistakes, from a feeling of inadequacy in a given situation" (68). Building women's sense of self, encouraging empowerment through movement, and being reminded of shared feelings of fear of failure can help to build individual and communal power.

The many circular movements in belly dance require letting go, a pertinent reminder that a circle is "without beginning or end, self-contained, perfect, and alone" (108). As we circle our hips, chest, head, wrists, we are reminded of our self-contained perfectness, of our individuality, and our connection with our own bodies. But belly dancing is about going within one's self while also connecting to what's outside oneself. We are reminded of this connection as we learn snake arms and other arm movements. As Al-Rawi writes, "the furthest point always remains an expression of the innermost" (89). We might consider how our expressions are communicated by ourselves and read by others. Al-Rawi reminds each of us to listen to ourselves and to listen to others, to listen to our body and beyond our body. Listening is an important feminist action. Too many of us like to talk, to be heard, and fail to listen to what others think. And too many of us fail to listen to ourselves, to our intuition or to our bodies.

There are many empowering messages that accompany the kinesthetic movements that we learn in belly dancing. As we focus on learning new movements, I remind students what Al-Rawi says, "remember that you are often biased in your self-criticism, that you see failures where an objective observer would never find fault" (68). This advice certainly applies to the way we might criticize ourselves as we dance, or engage in any kind of physical fitness program. But the feminist value goes deeper. In a culture where we are taught to always be judging and, thus, may worry about being judged, this advice reminds us that "outside observers" may be our allies. There is no need for the "catfights" that reality TV glorifies and Leora Tannenbaum critiques and illuminates.[17] And as we tend to think of bias as a problem that other people have, we might remember that we all have biases and we might work to examine and discard our biases. Letting go of bias and self-criticism (different from self-conscious self-criticism) may help us let go physically and emotionally.

Thus, Al-Rawi reminds us of the most important lesson; "before you can extend beyond yourself, you must first learn to know yourself" (138). This self-consciousness can lead to individual empowerment but more, it connects us outside ourselves since "to learn to know oneself is the basis for all understanding and love" (154). Feminism, women's studies, and fitness all have as a quality, if not a goal, a means toward self-love, self-consciousness, and a connection outside oneself. Feminism provides theory and political identity. Women's studies provides consciousness. And fitness provides release, expression, power.

Al-Rawi's guidance draws upon her belly dance education — growing up amongst a community of women who shared dance as celebration, connection, ritual, and expression — she translates for us, toward feminist fitness.

Fitness and Spirituality: Church and State of Mind

"Women's fitness as we know it truly is our newest form of patriarchal religion.... No wonder nobody trusts Jane Fonda anymore. Fitness is a rigid religion of style, as debilitating and oppressive for many as a corset."
— Alisa Valdés, "Ruminations of a Feminist Fitness Instructor" (31)

"I don't need yoga to be a religion. I need it to provide community. Community that acts consciously and pragmatically for the common good. Community that is not bankrupted by its exclusive consumer classism. Community that reaches out as much as it reaches in."
— Matthew Remski, "Modern Yoga Will Not Form a Real Culture Until Every Studio Can Also Double as a Soup Kitchen...." (110)

Valdés's comparison of fitness to a "patriarchal religion" is problematic in many ways. Her flippant reference to Jane Fonda shows a catty side of "feminism." Certainly the reasons why "nobody trusts Jane Fonda anymore" have something to do with Fonda's feminist politics, as well as her public persona. But this dig at Jane Fonda is only one of Valdés's arrogant judgments of other women — she also takes more than one shot at cheerleaders and at the whole of women in fitness. In her experience, if fitness is a "rigid religion of style," then she is only experiencing fitness in its most superficial forms, on its most superficial levels. While the comparison of certain kinds of fitness to a corset has its merits, and while fitness is oppressive in many of its mainstream, patriarchal incarnations (past and present), this limited way of looking at women's fitness discounts the many benefits — spiritual and otherwise that women glean from their fitness experiences within this patriarchal regime.

In contemporary women's lives, fitness and religion might seem to be at odds with each other. For instance, the "Ripped, Bikini-Clad Reverend," Rev. Dr. Amy Richter, writes about her struggle between training for and participating in physique competition at the Wisconsin State Fair and her work as an Episcopal priest. She writes, "I am usually more interested in what is going on inside a person than in what shows on the outside." This personal quandary is one facet, but the public perception is another. She continues, "this was a wholesome environment; still, I knew I couldn't share widely what I was doing." Because of previous, and sometimes continuing concerns, over women's ability to be priests, Richter feels that her role in fitness culture would not be a welcome aspect of her professional identity. She sums up the problem: "It has to do with having a woman's body," and she provides multiple examples of struggles with her body that members of her congregation have mentioned to her. Thus, much of her struggle centers around the required uniform for the competition: "What about when a priest wears a bikini? What if she complicates the picture by having sizable biceps or well-defined lats? Can 'buff' and 'holy' go together? 'Ripped' and 'reverend'? If the 'reverend' is a woman?"

Ultimately, she takes pride in her second-place win, and in the satisfaction of beating an amateur wrestler who placed third. She describes how she is announced as a priest when it is her turn on stage and how she proudly carries her trophy around the fair grounds. It is so flashy, she notes, that children stop her to ask her how she won such a fantastic trophy. Richter writes, "I wanted to say I won it ... for being a woman who is a priest with a really strong and healthy body. I wanted to tell them I won it for being brave, but that wasn't really true, because I hadn't been brave enough to tell the people it would be the biggest risk to tell." But the results of keeping this secret from her congregation are also a form of personal satisfaction for herself. She is empowered, perhaps, by the secret accomplishment as much as she is by the process of becoming "ripped." Her answer to the children who ask about her trophy: "'I got it for being myself.'"

For a woman priest, a fitness obsession is in conflict with her role, in part because of the emphasis it puts on her body. This is particularly true for something like Richter's passion — a display of chiseled muscles in as little clothing as possible. Even so, an April/May 2009 article, "Churches and Fitness — A Growing Trend," on the Faith & Fitness Magazine website. Author Rob Killen has interest in helping churches grow their fitness ministry. He outlines some of the evolution of fitness over the past 30 years and then argues that "churches all across America and throughout the world are adding fitness and recreation services as part of their ministry. Many churches currently have fitness facilities, and even more have fitness areas included in their future expansion plans." Churches are part of the progress of the fitness industry, Killen argues, placing them alongside other businesses that have incorporated fitness for their customers and employees, like hotels and corporate offices.

He also argues that there are plenty of reasons for churches to invest in faith ministry, despite those who think that fitness is not a responsibility of the church to its community. He explains these reasons: "church-goers are not as healthy as other people"; "complete well-being involves our physical bodies"; "fitness can serve as a great outreach tool"; and fitness can also provide "an alternative to church-goers who exercise elsewhere" and bolster a church's budget. The practical reasons of outreach and bolstering a budget appeal to the realities of the money and services it takes to serve a community of people; Killen also provides savvy, almost smarmy advice. Capture those who might be uncomfortable attending church services by "welcoming" them in through fitness. Establishing this "relationship" with them might result in getting them to join and serve the church. And, get your existing members to pay the church to provide fitness services instead of paying their money to places like the YMCA or gyms. More income will be generated by the church and this money will help to fund other aspects of the church in addition to the fitness.

Ultimately, Killen quotes scripture as reason to link fitness to church and concludes that:

> We glorify God by how we treat our physical body.... Once people begin to associate church as the one place they can always go to improve every area of their lives (spiritually, physically, mentally, and emotionally) regular church attendance on Sunday will grow, and more people will seek to become involved in other areas of your church ministry.

Certainly, Killen makes a convincing argument, particularly because his reasons include sound business as well as appeals to a more holistic approach to both ministry and fitness. And his goals of improving people's spiritual, physical, mental, and emotional lives are certainly worthy goals.[18] They are also goals that have a long history of religious fervor.

As James C. Wharton argues in *Crusaders for Fitness: The History of American Health Reformers*, the "levels of devotion, asceticism, and zeal" in early health crusaders can be "described as hygienic religion" (4). With hygiene as the foundation for all human progress (4), Wharton argues that "religious analogy has in fact commonly been used by health crusaders (and their detractors) to describe their missions" (4). Considering that only two pages later he argues that "most hygienic ideologists have espoused Christianity" (6), this religious analogy seems particularly fitting. This book is full of interesting information about the connections between religion, health, fitness, and diet as Wharton identifies the "major themes of health extremism as they evolved between 1830 and 1920" (11). The connections between this past history of, for instance, vegetarianism, physical education, a sound mind and body, and other elements deserve far more attention than I can give them here. But this history holds an important road map for radical reform for "present-day health reformers" (12).[19] Many of these influencers take the "self-help" angle, an approach that fits with the modern focus on the individual but also retains some of the roots of hygienic religion. This aspect of fitness speaks to spirituality and/or some other category that can't be explained by physical or mental categories alone. We look to health and fitness in a search for meaning.

* * *

Being non-religious, and actively defusing the religion of my rather liberal Presbyterian youth, only recently have I felt a spiritual connection to fitness, and I rarely describe my fitness routine or teaching as *spiritual*. It sounds off-putting. It sounds fake. It does not feel genuine. And because I have not embraced any kind of religion for a long time (if ever), and because I have mocked and critiqued other forms of spiritual enlightenment as much as I have avoided the subject of religion, considering anything as a spiritual endeavor puts me on guard. Mind and body are easy to grasp; soul, spirit, the power of the universe — these seem to require a leap of faith. I prefer to explore the edges — science-fictional excursions into the possibilities of the power of the universe and the possibilities of humankind. Sometimes fitness offers such possibilities.

Yoga is the fitness form most often associated with spirituality. As William J. Broad notes, yoga in the West has transitioned from ideas of magic and eroticism to health and fitness (11). These spiritual associations often keep people from trying yoga. They are afraid that it might be a dangerous spiritual line to balance on. But religion can drive some to skewed ideas like "Outstretched in Worship," featured briefly in the film *Yoga, Inc.* Similarly, Laurette Willis has created a "Christian ALTERNATIVE to Yoga," featured on her PraiseMoves website. Yoga poses are named things like "the standing cross" and "the altar" and scriptures are attached to the physical practice of yoga. This feels too forced to be a spiritual practice; it takes a deep, non-religiously-affiliated practice and stuffs it into a Christian box. Since the physical practice of yoga is only one aspect of the larger world of eight limbs of yoga and many incarnations of the physical, PraiseMoves is taking its agenda and layering it on top of movements that hold other significances. As one scrolls through the PraiseMoves website, the interpretations get more abstract and intense. Even for some Christians, the extreme Biblical interpretations of Willis are too much to take seriously.[20]

Yoga is also a resource for some Americans in a search for greater spiritual understanding. Some look a little too hard for spiritual meaning in fitness, hoping for some kind of transcendent epiphany when they attend yoga. In Elizabeth Gilbert's *Eat, Pray, Love*, a kind of spiritual crisis drives "One Woman's Search for Everything Across Italy, India and Indonesia." She remarks on the "happy coincidence that all these countries begin with the letter *I*" (3) as well as the ways in which her not-so-spiritual "wise-ass" friends make fun of what other kinds of *I*-countries she could have chosen. While she is looking for spiritual meaning, she is also looking for herself. Thus, the "I" theme is fitting. And while I personally find her voice to be overbearing and indulgent, Gilbert is certainly honest regarding her assumptions and short-comings. She also discovers some interesting and important connections between yoga and spirituality and some important insights about religion. For instance, she notes that our job is "to keep searching for the metaphors, rituals and teachers that will help [us] move ever closer to divinity" because "flexibility is just as essential for divinity as is discipline" (206). Despite a friend's cautions against it, Gilbert argues that we "have every right to cherry-pick when it comes to moving your spirit and finding peace in God.... You take whatever works from wherever you can find it, and you keep moving toward the light" (208). Markula reminds us that "the solution is not to switch from 'bad westernized' discourses to 'good' eastern philosophy and then blindly follow this new discourse" (73). Any kind of singular approach to a fitness philosophy is as problematic as any other kind of singular obsession.

We tread dangerous ground when we consider fitness as a spiritual practice though fitness certainly engages the body and the mind as well as feelings and experiences that are more difficult to quantify. The many traditions that influence fitness trends, moves, music, and practice can be used toward a variety of purposes and, then, sometimes can extract, skew, or steal, cultural traditions. We appropriate what is not ours toward individual enlightenment. We look for wisdom. We should be careful not to trample the source of our mental and physical movements. Respect is certainly one aspect of a feminist fitness, but feminist fitness spirituality is not simply a compilation of other (or "Othered") traditions, except as it is rooted in feminist traditions, ideologies, and practices. A feminist fitness spirituality takes root as it grows from theory and practice, but mostly from practice laced with theory. We find this in the ordered chaos of dance movements as well as in the straight and narrow of dominant fitness pursuits.

On the Run/On the Road/Walk It Off

"While weight reduction is a domestic activity, locked in the cupboards and kitchens of the home, exercise releases women onto the streets, gym and track — sites saturated in patriarchal histories and truths. Beyond low-fat cooking and the weigh in, feminism can run with fitness."
— Tara Brabazon, "Fitness Is a Feminist Issue" (79)

"My life story is embedded in the roads ... each neighborhood contains a story, a memory from a previous run, because the roads have become my journal. I am ever grateful for the ability to run and for the honor of sharing the joy of experiencing my body through a community of women (and men) athletes. I hope to still have the privilege of running when I am in my sixties and beyond...."
— Wendy Walter-Bailey, "If These Roads Could Talk: Life as a Woman on the Run" (149)

American culture keeps us on the run, so to speak. We are always moving, always going, but often also standing still at the same time. Women cannot outrun the pace of our lives; it's like we're on a treadmill that just keeps moving and as long as we are moving with it, we're in the game. We spin our wheels, sometimes going only where our imagination takes us.[21] We're also told to "walk it off," whether the "it" is an injury, a bad attitude, or the extra weight we carry. But running (or walking, or biking) for fitness might just help us to deal with that pace, maybe even slow it down. And maybe even find qualities that go beyond the obvious cardiovascular fitness benefits.

For those who are afraid to step into a gym for any variety of reasons — from feeling uncomfortable in the space to feeling uncomfortable in their bodies, from feeling intimidated by choreography to feeling clumsy and uncoordinated — running seems the logical cardiovascular choice. Thus, running is often the go-to fitness choice for women and men alike. It looks simple and no instructor or how-to manual are needed to get running. However, looks are deceiving; running can be far more complicated than putting one foot in front of the other despite the fact that it has been done since (conceivably) the beginning of human life and is even practiced without the modern amenity of shoes. But despite the lack of a need for specialized equipment, the popularity of running, like other sports and fitness pursuits, has inspired a plethora of gear from clothing and shoes to anti-chafing ointments to the irony-exuding shoes created for barefoot running.[22]

And there are many benefits to running. As Wendy Walter-Bailey argues, "running might allow us to clear our minds, manage our weight, deal with stress, and raise our self esteem" (145). Running is certainly a favorite fitness activity (not mine!) and it became popular in the 1970s, in part as a result of Cooper's research. Running is the most accessible way to build cardiovascular health — no equipment is needed, no other people are needed, and it can be done at any time. It also has the added benefit of the "runner's high," a phenomenon that gets a full chapter of Gina Kolata's attention: "Is There a Runner's High?" Running is also a solitary form of exercise, a benefit many people cherish. And, yet, running is also a very public form of fitness. As such, women may be vulnerable in their pursuits of this form of fitness.

In *Women and Exercise*, Jacqelyn Allen-Collinson cannot separate the fitness activity from the dangers of public space, and before she begins to outline a "feminist phenomenology of female running" she reviews the "extensive analysis" of "the social structuring" of public space. She writes, "running in public space undoubtedly renders women (and also in some contexts, men) vulnerable to harassment — verbal and on occasions physical, even assault" (289). She relates her experiences of such harassment while she also examines data from research projects "in relation to my lived-body experiences of the paradoxes and tensions of the vulnerable but also powerful female running body" (281). Her concern is less with running as a fitness pursuit and more with "women's sporting embodiment" (281). She concludes, in part, "the paradoxical, contradictory nature of exercising in public space.... On the one hand, the negative structures of experience loom large.... On the other hand, the positive elements include the experience of empowerment, social agency, resistance, bodily power, strength and sensory pleasure" (288). These benefits are less often considered in relationship to running; this activity is often shrunken down to its lowest common denominator — running is a good (cardio) workout.

Allen-Collinson's feminist-phenomenological perspective does, in fact, "generate fresh research insights" (293), particularly regarding the carnal, 'fleshy,' lived ... moving, sweating" female body. Ultimately, however, her study hinges upon the her own lived-body experience, a powerful site for analysis if not also an isolated, singular "lifeworld ... of a female distance runner" (293). Many of the same experiences she describes can be found with less danger in another lifeworld or with a different image of the female distance runner. As Walter-Bailey discovers, running can be more powerful in community. She notes: "I did not anticipate the way my life would change when I started running with other women" (146). This community provides more than just safety; it provides a space to work out more than just the body.

And we don't have to be on the run to enjoy many of these same benefits — enjoying nature, clearing our heads, managing our weight, and finding community among women. Many people think that they cannot get the same fitness benefits from walking as they can from running and this is, perhaps, partly true. You have to spend more time walking to burn the same number of calories, but caloric expenditure is only one measure. As Gina Kolata notes, the ancient Greeks actually advocated walking for exercise and a balance of exercise and food for health. (31) Walking is low-impact but it doesn't have to be low-intensity; and walking can tone your legs, hips, and abdominals in different ways than running can. Running jars the back and the knees and puts a lot of pressure on the feet and ankles. Walking minimizes this stress and with the addition of walking poles, an upper-body workout can be added. Moreover, as Marlene Jensen explains, "Walking alone is exercise. Walking with friends, especially women friends, can be an enriching and transformative experience " (151). This kind of friendship is similar to the kind of friendship that Walter-Bailey builds with her group of runners: "there is a sisterhood among my running partners and me ... there is a special bond that I have not found anywhere else" (147), she writes.

With a group of walkers Jensen discovers the power that walking in community can provide. "Our walks were a combination of a family and neighborhood news network, group therapy, brainstorming, a workout, and, mostly, a special daily connection that celebrated the details of our lives. We were a walking example of contemporary women's history" (152). Walter-Bailey recognizes these benefits as well but in a sport that can be highly competitive, like running, she notes, "rather than compete against each other in a race, or even during a workout, our goal is to lift and encourage" (147). And this support is bigger than just a "you go girl!" She continues, "that all women's victories are supported, not only those who, somehow, fit into the standards of a patriarchal, capitalist system, is at the heart of our mission" (147). And this support goes beyond the personal, individual kind of support women give each other as they run. "... we run for all the women in our community, and we provide our money and our services to all kinds of organizations for women" (147). While the specifics of such philanthropy are omitted, the spirit of such support is alive and well. These ideals have been embodied in the organization Girls on the Run, a non-profit organization where "running is used to inspire and motivate girls, encourage lifelong health and fitness, and build confidence through accomplishment." But the focus of Girls on the Run is not simply on running or on exercise; Girls on the Run is "dedicated to creating a world where every girl knows and activates her limitless potential and is free to boldly pursue her dreams." Running certainly has more potential than its "simple," linear nature implies.

* * *

Alone or with friends, outside, or on the treadmill, running and walking can have many benefits. For me, running is a painful, boring experience and the treadmill is the worst-case-scenario workout choice. Running, walking, and biking all have a "straight and narrow" quality to them. They are linear and predictable and the body's motion is always, consistently the same. They all cover distance and are also modes of travel. Walking and running are rigidly structured by distance rather than time; if you get there, you know you have to get back. If you get a flat tire, you've got to fix it. Unless, of course, you are on a treadmill or stationary bike; if this is the case you can choose distance, time, or even terrain as your measure. To improve, a walker or runner or cyclist has to compete with time, the same distance in a shorter amount of time or a more difficult geography. These aspects of time, distance, and terrain are beneficial workout markers to some exercisers but, especially metaphorically, these are undesirable qualities to some. For instance, I can lose track of time in a cardio dance class; the class is over and sometimes I haven't even glanced at the prominently-displayed clock. While walking on the treadmill, I watch every second tick away and it is torture to get to a 30 minute mark. My walking (never running and rarely biking outside of transportation needs) is recreational; it has the side benefit of fitness and brings some variety and outdoor air to my fitness life. I hike and backpack and walk my dog. Only rarely do I feel the urge to run, to be unfettered and to feel the wind rush past my moving body. Then, I go for a run in my head and the urge fades. My body thanks me. I swear I will never take up running. To each her own. And then one day I miss my morning workout and I really need to blow off some steam. I find that maybe running is not so unenjoyable when it provides cold air in my lungs and an ache in my legs. The quiet, peaceful early evening, a brief "warm" spell in the middle of winter, a sense of freedom, are all signs that maybe I am not as opposed to running as I think I am. It's an activity I can appreciate from, or at, a distance. It is a movement that can help us find freedom ... and transformation.

Creative/Critical: Contradictions and Possibilities

"The cheerleaders never came to our [cross-country] meets because they were watching football. Being a runner was the first time (maybe not exactly) I embraced an 'otherness' and a disdain for the mainstream."
— Marcia Woodard, "The Gymnastics Group" (97).

With the popularity of running as a fitness choice, it seems counterintuitive that one would find an "otherness" in her identity as a runner. And yet, this statement illustrates at least two things. Women continue to be marginalized in their sports and fitness choices despite feminist gains. And, being a runner can engender an oppositional stance despite its "straight and narrow" properties. Fitness, generally, does not seem to be the space where "otherness" or "disdain for the mainstream" exist. We assume women are jumping around to look good for the patriarchy; they are losing weight to fit an impossible standard of the perfect body portrayed by the media. And yet fitness can teach us to question the mainstream and can build a resistance to those negative messages better than the standard academic lecture or clever advertising campaign might be able to. We might not consider that running or other fitness pursuits would help to develop a critical consciousness; however, fitness is ripe for feminist consciousness-raising, community-building, and critical analysis. Fitness, like life, is full of contradictions. Contradictions are reality and fitness aids our navigation.

Just as fitness is often seen as an activity that is counter to feminist agendas, it is also not often included in the realm of the creative arts. Further, this creative realm provides new kinds of feminist critical endeavors and creative expression. Some of this creativity is illustrated through the poems and creative nonfiction in *My Life at the Gym* and I follow this model — and extend it; in *Women and Fitness in American Culture* the creative/critical are fused and flexed. Through poetry as well as in the structure and methods of my work here, a mirror and meld of the classroom and the studio.

In her piece in *Home Girls Make Some Noise*, Chyann L. Oliver describes the importance of critical/creative approaches and merging art, academia, and activism. She writes:

... I have a unique writing style; I fuse poetry with scholarly/critical essay. I believe that it is crucial that knowledge be accessible to many people and in many forms. I use the combination of poetry and scholarly/critical essay to further my commitment to rejecting the activist/academic dichotomy because poetry/theatre, which is often viewed as activist and artistic, and non-academic, are theory, and should be validated as such.... As a Black female artist and academic, my duty is to bridge that gap and fight for all of our work to be recognized as valid without being apologetic for what we as scholar-activists do [251].

Oliver is coming from a very different place than I am, artistically and culturally; however, her theorizing here opens up possibilities for merging scholarship, art, and activism in new ways. The way she views and moves her work speaks to the ways in which I navigate my own "dichotomies" and merge scholarship, art, and activism.

* * *

As my ideas about feminist fitness developed — in theory and practice — I also began to think about these ideas in terms of "the critical and the creative," a submission category for the 2010 National Women's Studies Association (NWSA) conference on the theme of "Difficult Dialogs II." The call for submissions refers to a number of seminal works by feminists of color, including *This Bridge Called My Back*, works that "refused the false divide between creative expression and theoretical analysis." I began to think about how my work in fitness could be better understood by considering this false divide and the ways in which my fitness work involved both critical and creative work in both academic and fitness contexts.

In its call for "examinations of the epistemological and political dimensions of creativity in many forms," these many forms were left open, "not limited to filmmaking, new media technologies, narrative, and the fine and performing arts," the more traditional of the non-traditional arts. While fitness is, perhaps, not the first art we might think of, it certainly speaks to a certain "way of knowing" as well as the other work of academic feminists — teaching, researching, and activism — as well as our hope to resist and "intervene in dominant/hegemonic stories and histories." In this call I saw the possibility to connect my life in academia with my life in the fitness studio. Certainly fitness is a knowledge that has "not been fully realized within women's studies." I submitted the following abstract.

"Feminist Fitness: The Critical/Creative Through Power, Pleasure, and Movement":

I refuse the "false divide between creative expression and theoretical analysis" and my creative expression resists the false binary between mind and body, the academy and the community. This creative expression — a feminist fitness class — is designed to empower women and promote both creative physical movement and the movement of feminist consciousness. This workshop draws from my 10 years as a fitness instructor as well as from my feminist scholarship in cultural theory and popular culture. It blends the critical and the creative by offering a unique experience of music, dance, and feminist ideas disguised in a workout. The movement provides opportunity for experiences of power and pleasure, connections with other women, exploration of feminist ideas, and freedom of movement — a layered experience of the critical and the creative.

This workshop is a version of an event that I hold at my local YMCA in conjunction with Women's History month. It is also connected to my women's studies 101 classes where students read about belly dancing and learn the movements to give creative complement to their critical studies. Depending upon the time available for this workshop I can adjust what is usually about 1.5 hours of a dance class. Ideally, I would have 1.5 hours for the activity portion of the workshop and 45 minutes to an hour for a brief presentation of the critical theory behind this workshop and a critical discussion of questions like: "how can women's studies more fully engage the creative as a way of knowing?"

Because of time constraints, I offered an abbreviated feminist fitness class with some introduction and some discussion after we danced. While my abstract appealed to those who were organizing the conference, my workshop description is what appeared in the conference program, right alongside the more traditional examples of academic panels.

Feminist Fitness: The Critical/Creative Through Power, Pleasure, and Movement. Experience a fitness class that brings together the critical and the creative combining feminist ideas and music with movements that blend belly dancing, hip hop, and modern dance as well as yoga and the Nia technique to create a fun, powerful, and empowering workout. This is an interactive, activity-driven workshop so please be prepared to move but no dance or fitness experience required! While we explore the creative and critical through our individual and group physical movement we will also consider how fitness might be a site of resistance and how the creative allows us to intervene in dominant/hegemonic stories, histories, and ideologies.

The workshop drew about 25 people — far more than I expected — and if I had been prepared to pursue this work rather than just present it, I could have gathered some important feedback. But it was also nice to simply share my work as it had developed up to that point. Everyone was engaged and even enthusiastic about the fitness dance that we did. Afterward we had a lively discussion, and I was inspired to continue to develop my work in and out of academia.

* * *

The critical and creative are deeply intertwined in the realm of feminist fitness. This creative/critical methodology/pedagogy requires awareness and flexibility — the ability to combine a variety of approaches for a variety of people, to make them feel comfortable. It requires a base of knowledge — kinesthetic, feminist, practical, social — and the ability to apply this knowledge toward myriad goals. It requires innovation rooted in safe, proven techniques, and the ability to deliver the creative in a collective fitness space. It requires a critical eye and an awareness of difference.

The most overlooked creative endeavors are those of fitness instructors. Fitness is my creative outlet and I find that my choreography helps me connect my mind and my body with and through music and movement. Creating fitness choreography is no different from any other art. As Amalia Mesa-Bains argues, "art is inherently a social practice. It's a social act, and it's embedded in one's relationship to a larger world" (94). There is an element of activism as my choreography is created consciously, in an effort to intervene in negative body images through positive movement. The creation and execution of choreography and instruction reaches out and hopes to transform from conception to construction to execution to reflection, mixing the creative with the critical.

Unfortunately, the critical often scares people away. The language is unfamiliar. When looking for fitness, people seem to be more focused on standard results. When asking for my mom's opinion of a draft of a class description, she said I should add something about burning calories or sculpting sexy muscles. *People like that kind of thing.* Without the familiar results-based language people would be unsure and might not take the risk, she thought. She wasn't wrong.

The creative also scares people away. Upon my first encounter with Nia, I did not attend class because I feared it was too New-Agey; I heard the instructor lit candles and burned incense. My description for Power, Pleasure, and Movement also intimidated people — it is an unbranded, unpredictable fitness form. As my mother also reminded me, pleasure implies the carnal enjoyment that must not be found in fitness spaces where "no pain, no gain" still reigns. Perhaps Americans are too accustomed to standardization. If we want our fitness like we want our fast food, the irony overflows. Alternatives to Zumba, like Nia, for instance, are akin to "crunchy granola." The mainstream doesn't have the stomach or the taste buds for it. Those of us pushed to the edges have to fight to keep fitness creative and find ways to bring out its critical aspects as well. Such work pushes us to the edges of fitness and begs for a re-centering.

Four

Edges/Bodies and Minds

Exploring the Edges

Fitness is glossy images
and perfect ratios,
sculpted bodies and restricted eating,
pounding the pavement
gasping for air
muscle aches —
— inside/out
motivation

The edges of fitness skirt
the personal and political,
bind and recombine.

Fitness is love
and balance
agile bodies and free movement
pulsating beat
purging the soul
stretching, flexing —
— mind/body/self
motivation

The edges of fitness swirl
making inside out,
reflect and redefine.

* * *

In this section I pull no punches. The edges of fitness are sharp and they keep many of us away — away from the gym, away from ourselves — just as they keep many of us cycling through the same issues, repeating old patterns. The issues manifest in our bodies; they refuse to leave our minds. The issues manifest in our minds; they refuse to leave our bodies. Only movement, away

135

from one space and into another, can redefine the edge. Fitness can help to let those things go, to seek new things, to live in the present and prepare for the unknown, shifting future. As I explore the edges of my own life, other edges emerge as well. Secrets become shared experience and lose the weight they once held. Legacies and expectations become the power to see through the surface of things. The skewed mirror that society holds up to our faces, telling us we are too young, too old, too fat, too dark, too uptight, too free, takes up new angles to its reflections. It fogs over. It shatters and we search for new measures.[1] We recognize that the mind is a necessary component of fitness and that the mind/body connection is a powerful tool in a search for self and the challenges of daily life.

The edges are abrupt and drop suddenly.

But fitness is about balancing the mind and body. Regaining composure after teetering on the edge.

The edges provide strict definitions and solid lines.

But, fitness is feeling good and being okay with your body. It's about learning to see through damaging mainstream definitions — of gender, of age, of skin color, of body size or type. It's about finding what works and what fits, redefining and drawing new flexible lines.

The edges cut and try to tear us down.

But, fitness on the edge is about love — for self and others. It's about acceptance and freedom and empowerment and letting go.

At the edges we are not alone.

Cultural Appropriations and Cross-Cultural Connections

> "It cannot really be said that belly dancing is the product of one particular culture or tribe; it is a mixture, carried by a century-old knowledge, that has developed within certain social and historical circumstances."
>
> — Rosina Al-Fawi, *Grandmother's Secrets* (42)

One of the side effects of both the art of fitness (as a collage of moves and styles) and the character of the industry (as a pre-packaged, cool-hunter), is the appropriation of the traditions — the music and movements — of historically oppressed peoples. This is dangerous territory — walking the line of appropriation — but all forms of fitness evolve from other forms by incorporating movements and styles that already overlap from one form to another. Classic fitness moves combine with any variety of dance, sport, martial arts, and any other form of movement that can be adapted into the fitness realm. Any cultural form is inspiration for fitness movement. Sometimes this borrowing is done consciously, thoughtfully; sometimes it is coincidental or unconscious. Sometimes it is reverential to its origin, and sometimes it is insulting. And it all depends upon contexts and perspectives. While dance is infinite in its organic, artistic nature, there is a base of movements that any dancer/mover/artist draws from. Movements from belly dancing are recognizable in Hula dance and some other indigenous dance forms as well as in Hip-Hop dance. Yoga has a finite set of postures with endless variation. It also varies greatly from school to school, style to style, instructor to instructor, and the physical practice of yoga is only one of eight traditional branches. There is sameness and difference woven tightly. Perhaps, then, fitness is something that brings people together across difference?

To illustrate the hybrid, flexible, malleable nature of fitness movement is not to excuse any of its cultural appropriations. Certainly the chain of influence throughout the ages of the development of dance (around the world, formally and informally), and the decades of formal development of the field of fitness, would be difficult to separate, delineate, measure, and weigh. To extract "Other" and "Othered" traditions from fitness would be impossible. And yet it is certainly easy to see the more extreme side of cultural appropriations in the fitness industry. Capitalist markets combined with patriarchal expectations of women's bodies combined with American ideologies of competition, survival of the fittest, and individual responsibility combined with white supremacy and a tradition of violence and imperialism against nonwhite and/or "third world" and/or terrorist bodies, makes for a volatile mixture of fitness propaganda. While more explorations of the individual level of experiences concerning race and fitness are necessary for a deeper and broader understanding, in this section I am more concerned with the structural level of (media) representation. How can we understand the fine line between incorporation and appropriation, inspiration and misrepresentation, celebration and pandering? Considering a few examples illustrates the complicated nature of race, culture, and fitness.

American fitness programs and trends cross racial and ethnic lines; they also travel across borders and fulfill their own niches in other places in the world. For instance, in 2010, *IDEA Fitness Journal* featured a column called "World Beat" that "explores the activities and fitness trends of IDEA members around the world." Contributing editor, Alexandra Williams, explores Kazakhstan and Thailand; and another contributing editor, April Durrett, considers Spain and Venezuela, for instance. Each column considers fitness in its particular context, interviewing fitness professionals and highlighting trends.

For the most part, these columns consider the kinds of exercise that are also prevalent in the U.S., and are regularly featured in *IDEA Fitness Journal*: group fitness, mind/body fitness, and personal training. These forms are also popular outside the U.S., and the "World Beat" column shows how other countries have similar trends that vary according to custom, economic conditions, interest, ability, and other factors that differ from place to place. These columns also highlight to varying degrees: gender differences, cultural traditions that complement and influence Western forms of fitness, and the involvement of government in promoting fitness and health. These columns explore the cultural attitude toward fitness as a trend, a form of employment, and a means toward culturally desirable goals like looking good or living well spiritually. Most often, the column ends on an optimistic note; more people are, we hope, coming to understand the importance of fitness. More than anything else, these columns offer a glimpse at cultural differences while highlighting the ways in which fitness — as a concept and activity — crosses borders and evolves. These columns are cultural tours and cross-cultural connections rather than sustained analyses of what makes fitness unique to a certain place. Such an approach is what we should expect from an industry trade journal. But expecting, and accepting as an adequate consideration of Othered spaces, are two different things.

Just as American fitness ideas travel to other locations around the world, cultural traditions and local incarnations travel to the U.S. as well. The Masala Bhangra Workout, for instance, created by Sarina Jain (who is described as the "Jane Fonda of India"), is described as:

> an exercise dance routine that modernizes the high-energy folk dance of Bhangra by blending traditional Bhangra dance steps and the exhilaration of Bollywood (Hindi film) moves, seen recently in the Oscar-winning film *Slumdog Millionaire*! This unique dance mixes cardiovascular [fitness] with fun, and is suitable for participants of all ages and fitness levels.

Drawing upon the popularity of the most widely-known film to feature Indian characters, as well as the iconic status of Jane Fonda, The Masala Bhangra Workout is a dance aerobics incarnation with ethnic dance at its roots, delivered in the American aerobics vessel. This workout crosses cultures and embodies difference and sameness. It shares some qualities with the more well-known aerobics dance form, Zumba.

The famous creator of Zumba, Alberto "Beto" Perez is, in many ways, a poster boy for cross-cultural connections. He is from Columbia and got his start with Zumba in Miami; now Zumba is taught "from Canada to China." In an interview with *Reader's Digest*, Perez notes that "working with other cultures" has been "a challenge," citing an example of bringing Zumba to Thailand. He also notes that he is now producing music and plans to bring "more international beats to the mix." Now a success around the world, Beto's story is recounted as an American success story. One day he forgot his regular music, grabbed a tape of Spanish-language music from his car, and innovated movement. And Zumba was born. Despite his lack of English-language skills, he was able to bring Zumba to the U.S. As a 2009 article in *Reader's Digest* explains: "the fitness and dance instructor simply wanted to bring his workout classes to America. But with little money and even less English, he couldn't get fitness-center managers to watch his Latin-dance-inspired videos." But an infomercial went straight to the people.

Many stories highlight Beto's difference as well as his success — measured through popularity and profit (illustrated through numbers in the millions). Now the creative director, Perez did not grow Zumba by himself but had the help of people with the business know-how, even if they didn't have the funding. As *Reader's Digest* explains, when funding opportunities fell through after 9–11, they made an infomercial "which sold about a million DVDs in six months." And from there, people wanted to become Zumba instructors like Beto. "Since the first workshop, in 2003, the partners, based in Hollywood, Florida, have created a global community of instructors." The price of being a Zumba instructor, particularly compared to other fitness instructor programs, is relatively inexpensive — about $250 for training and a license. The global branding brings in the participants in droves and the required training is minimal — one day with no required follow-up or demonstration of skills. For $30 a month, instructors get a network, advertising, and regular choreography with very little investment. And almost a decade later, Zumba continues to draw crowds.

While Perez certainly has talent and a product with mass appeal, his "Otherness" has been key in the appeal of his Latin dance product in the U.S. His product has authenticity, even when it is watered down by individual instructors. The name itself symbolizes the Otherness in tandem with mainstream popularity. This appeal is similar to one of those American contradictions regarding race. For instance, racism creates a hierarchy of color, light to dark, that persists in the U.S., within racialized U.S. communities, and around the world. Women in Africa and India, for instance, use skin-lightening products like Fair and Lovely to lighten their skin while white Americans spend millions tanning to make themselves darker (and, thus, more "attractive").[2] Likewise, Americans discount much of the expertise and knowledge that comes from people of color, particularly when it comes to issues of race, while imbuing bodies of color with special significance when it comes to particular knowledge or pursuits, like Zumba. For instance, Shaun T's *Hip Hop Abs* and other such incarnations of this famous fitness figure (pun intended) appeal to, and are marketed to, white audiences who can understand *Hip Hop*

Abs as more "authentic" if it comes from a brown body. Shaun T's *Hip Hop Abs* video even begins with a little rap about working your abs and is full of lively, encouraging banter. As these aspects reinforce stereotypes related to race, they also simultaneously challenge and support conceptions of what constitutes a fit body (six-pack abs) or a fitness practice (workout video).[3]

Simultaneously combating and inadvertently reinforcing, racial categories, Yoga celebrities, Rodney Yee and Wai Lana are, in part, celebrated through a kind of Orientalist assumption of the superiority of Asian mysticism.[4] Yoga has an association with the East making such Asian influences feel more "natural" to unaware Americans, even if Asia is a large, diverse set of countries. Similarly, yoga retreats to India as well as to Mexico or Costa Rica hold an appeal of authenticity as "Other." A complicated kind of cultural appropriation is at work in these examples and perhaps someone less cynical (or less informed) might see these as being innocent multicultural examples. Maybe they are, but they are also examples of essentialized racial representations; they rely upon popular stereotypes and do not challenge structural inequalities. Even so, there is some opportunity for cross-cultural connection here. The common denominator is fitness.

Musical connections might be some of the best ways to see the cross-cultural connections in the world of fitness. Musical genius Michael Franti (of Spearhead) is a well-known yogi who appears in many documentaries (for instance, *Yoga Is*) and interviews on the subject, and can also sometimes be found offering up his talents through live music for yoga classes. He's also the co-founder (with Carla Swanson) of Stay Human, an apparel company that has recently opened Soulshine Bali, a yoga retreat center. Franti's work includes being Ambassador for CARE, a organization that works to "fight global poverty by empowering girls and women to bring lasting change to their communities." He also founded the annual Power to the Peaceful festival and participates in yoga fundraisers as well as many other efforts that combine yoga, business, music, art, community, and social justice. On the Stay Human website Franti explains:

> As a conscious musician and dedicated yogi, I have traveled the world practicing in beautiful yoga studios, dirty backstage dressing rooms, hotel conference rooms and grassy fields at festivals. I've been inspired by dozens of teachers and have met amazing people in the yoga community in every city I've visited. It's exciting to witness the exponential worldwide growth of yoga and the way it inspires people to become more present to themselves, their communities and to the planet.[5]

Franti has the opportunity to travel widely and his ability to connect with "the yoga community" speaks to the nature of this community as "transcendent"—it crosses, time and place as well as region and culture.[6] Franti also embodies cross-cultural connections through his mixed-race heritage and identity as well as his soulful, political, playful, loving, moving music. Franti's music moves people, literally and figuratively. He recognizes "All the Freaky People" and reminds us to "Stay Human." He celebrates life, critiques culture and politics, spreads love, builds community, and challenges oppression. My students — in the academic classroom and in the fitness studio — are inspired by his music.

Another musical artist, rapper, and yogi, MC Yogi, also makes cross-cultural connections by fusing Hip Hop and Hindu myths and mantras. On his album, *Elephant Power* (2008), he tells stories of Krishna, Shiva, Parvarti, and Genesh, for instance. It's an easy way to sneak some "Othered" cultures' stories into an unsuspecting yoga class. MC Yogi's music is also useful for class instruction. "Chakra Beat Box," for instance, provides sounds, words, and a beat to match movements to; it allows the concepts of chakras — or energy centers — to be introduced in a non-threatening and enlightening (and fun!) way. We can feel the benefits of the chakra-balancing movements set to music. With *Pilgrimage* (2012), MC Yogi provides a number of songs that work well into a yoga class. "Temple Light" provides a focus on the ribcage, and I can emphasize movement, stillness, inner light, or breathing through the lyrics and music. I use MC Yogi's (and Franti's) music in dance classes as well as yoga classes. MC Yogi's bonus tracks "Give Love" and its remix provide an upbeat tempo and an opportunity to share movement and space as well as love.

While there are many more facets of fitness and race to explore critically, in and out of academia, there is the possibility to bridge cultures through movement.[7] Essentially, this is what María Lugones suggests when she argues that "travelling to someone's 'world' is a way of identifying with them because travelling to their 'world' we can understand *what it is to be them and what it is to be ourselves in their eyes*" (401, author's emphasis). The space of the yoga studio or a dance or fitness studio is a "world," and we explore it as we travel across cultures in embodied ways. As Al-Rawi argues in *Grandmother's Secrets*, "By experiencing unfamiliar movements, a woman can allow her body to break through cultural norms" (viii). This can act as a "bridge towards greater understanding and respect for women who come from other cultures" (viii). These kinds of bridges are akin to Lugones' "'world'-travelling" and have been explored in academia through works like the seminal *This Bridge Called My Back: Radical Writings by Women of Color* and other works, most often by feminists of color and queer feminists. There is always more work to be done in terms of understanding cross-cultural connections, but it is also important to remember that the ability to "break through cultural norms" is, in many ways, a prerequisite for building such bridges. The body is a starting point.

Sketches: Bodies, Faces, and Names: Part and Whole, the People Who Take Fitness Classes

> "It [aerobics] is not a reification of femininity, but one of the few places where women of different ages, classes, ethnicities and educational levels can meet, mingle and talk. Under the lycra, beyond the beat and removed from the repetition is a diverse collective of women who build friendships, discuss their lives and think about the world."
> — Tara Brabazon, "Fitness Is a Feminist Issue" (79)

They say thank you. Perfect. That's just what I needed. They slip out five minutes early or arrive five minutes late. They resist change. They greet newcomers. They go with the flow. They guard their chosen space and accommodate new additions. They hide in t-shirts, find sparkles at the thrift store, and customize their shoes. Sisters, friends, mothers and daughters. Strangers. Acquaintances. Partners. Community.

Names don't often stick unless I write them, say them, and connect the name with a face and a characteristic. I learn names better when I observe other people calling someone's name. In the group exercise room, people come and go. I learn names by eavesdropping on conversations, through sporadic introductions, by repeating a name over and over to myself and vowing to make it stick. Faces and bodies flow — they mix with other places, other times, other faces. Faces and bodies stick. I look forward to the variations, adaptations, missed steps, ebb and flow — the dependable, steady flow of regulars.

Pat always wears the same blue leotard bottoms. She always thanks me for class. She always smiles and, when I move away, she says good-bye to me with chocolate.

Gwethalyn's strong shapely calves. People tell me she has lost a lot of weight. Later, I find out she survived breast cancer. Twice. Somewhere, she found fitness. She rarely misses class and always has the same spot. The instructors look to her when they forget the choreography. She knows all the moves.

Tessa moves with ease. That's not how she sees herself. But she slips right into the groove. The more she comes to class, the more she begins to believe. (She cries when she reads this.)

After attempting headstands, Kathy tells me of her shrunken brain tumor. She wonders if she should be doing headstands. (Of course not!) The pieces fall into place. But she is so strong. She hikes and kayaks and works out regularly. She is a survivor. But she complains all the time. Then she tires of "gentle yoga"; she leaves to look for something more challenging. She finds Group Core. She continues to complain about my class, even after not taking it for a couple of years.

Ellie sets up her step in the back corner. She steps at her pace. She complains about everything but she always comes back.

Sue greets every new person. She complains about the hard work, but there is no substance — only humor — in her whining. She always thanks me for class. She heard me lament my love of smoothies and my lack of a blender in my temporary apartment. The next class, she brought me her blender in a brown paper bag. I returned it full of chocolate.

Ali is often the only man in class and he is a long-time participant in step. He wears black spandex shorts and a black t-shirt. His chunks of silver jewelry seem weightless. He laughs at the idea that people think he must be gay but he never attempts to correct their opinions. He likes when I play "Blue Monday" and he rarely misses class. He is a professor in some kind of science field and a vegetarian. One day his wife takes my yoga class. I see him sometimes walking his dog.

I hope that Jade knows how beautiful she is. She moves well, and she has been coming to class consistently. I know she isn't seeing the weight loss results that other members are seeing. Like mine, her body likes to hold on to weight. She disappears. Temporarily?

Margaret's glasses sit by her yoga mat when we're in down dog. She and Elsie never miss Sunday yoga. Sometimes they are my only participants. They are always so grateful for class, and they support my "feminist fitness" endeavors and bring Nia to our gym. We enjoy our time together. When I move just an hour North, they shower me with gifts.

Tamara shows me her spiral tattoo — acquired when she discovered women's studies. An instant connection. She's in grad school studying art therapy. She's here tonight for belly dance fitness. I see her only a few more times. I hope she finds her way back. But so many people disappear, fade in and fade out.

The weight melts off of Crystal. She works at it and switches up her workout to get the results she wants and feels she needs. She worries about the jiggle, which is all the loose skin that remains. The whole is not yet the sum of the parts. I hope she is staying healthy in her expectations; I keep her on my radar. When she tells me I dance beautifully, I laugh off the compliment. And then I remind myself I need to stop doing that; I need to be able to take a compliment. I need to believe her. So, she reminds me to believe.

Betty's spot is in the front right corner. No one would take Betty's spot;

she has earned it. She reminds us. At 76, she comes to class consistently, at least 5 or more times a week. She has leotard/tight combos in a variety of colors — all green, all purple, stripes. Often a sequined headband or something sparkly. She likes the step class and the Group Groove the best. She hates when "they" do kickboxing. She tolerates my belly dance moves. She complains all the time. Sometimes she has a coughing fit. She is sick (she reminds me) and exercise keeps her going. (So does the complaining, I think.) She gives us chocolates — the ones with the positive sayings inside — and sometimes oranges after class.

Keri's daughter, Sarah, is seven years old and she practices belly dancing at home. Sometimes she dances with us. Other time she watches, reads, giggles, wiggles, runs, twirls. She brings out the mats for us and hangs on her favorite class members. Keri tells me this is the only fitness class where she feels at home. And, no doubt, having Sarah there makes it even more welcoming.

When Keri's life gets hectic, Mary and her daughter, Rachel (also age seven), start coming to class. Rachel informs maintenance when the disco ball needs to be fixed (and it gets done!), and she dances the whole class. My favorite part is when she nods her head with purpose leading into the hook for "Girl on Fire" by Alicia Keyes. I work this head nod into my choreography.

Randy is often the only man in Group Groove (and Cardio Mix). He's a bit off beat but full of anticipatory enthusiasm. He works hard to learn the moves. He works out hard in the weight room and does cardio on his own in addition to class. He works the room with high fives and always answers the "how are we doing?" call loudly and affirmatively. Class just isn't the same without him; he brings the energy for us all. His work schedule gets in the way.

Lisa has her Ashtanga yoga routine. It does not change; it develops, deepens. She follows it with purpose, grace. For me Ashtanga is stultifying; for her, routine and satisfying.

The ladies at Val's studio giggle and ask where I'll be standing. They are fearless, trusting, accepting. I fill in for Val, half-asleep at 8:00 on a Saturday morning. They jump right in and try out my stuff. They have fun. They ask if I'll be back. I will be, but things change.

Teen and pre-teen girls have started to take my classes. (I wish that I had found fitness classes when I was their age.) They inspire me and I wish I had more time to create classes just for girls. They make requests sometimes, but their attendance is inconsistent.

Nancy always has a smile on her face and braces on her knees. Bunny is focused. Kathy groans in anticipation. Katie is all strength and grace. Christine and Lisa make it look easy.

The Freys are loyal, passionate. Jim, a retired college professor who climbs mountains, always gives positive feedback. He jokes about his inability to give up competition. I'm working on him. Marcia gives updates on the growing brood of grandchildren. She brings me just enough fudge for the holidays. They miss class for vacations and family visits, little else. The front of the room feels empty when they're gone.

Patricia drives everyone crazy. Complains, again (too hot/too cold, too dark/too light). Does her own thing, front and center. She moves too much or not at all. Too often her disability and persona keep her isolated in a full room. She talks to herself, sometimes yells. Sometimes barks. She loves dance. She explores dance with a passion and politely asks me questions about belly dancing. She doesn't like to move her hips and never does the chest circles, but she tells me that taking belly dancing has helped her dance more generally. I give her a ride home sometimes on cold nights. Suddenly, she disappears.

After class Lydia asks me/tells me that my Just Dance class really increased her self confidence. *Is it possible that it could do that?* Her face lights up; she attended only a couple of classes and she was surprised by their effect. This is exactly what I try to tell people, but sometimes you have to just feel it.

Through the crack in the door, the Navy ROTC's jacks and grunts infiltrate our yoga space as we breathe into our cat/cows. Dorian mocks them, "and breathe 2–3–4"; we laugh. She takes yoga to her bunny, creating new poses. Pat the bunny. Mama cave.

Judith is focused, controlled.

Diana is serious, relaxed.

A new woman comes to cardio kickboxing. She's full of energy, clearly experienced. She exudes joy throughout class and yells "yes!" when I ask if we can feel our abdominals working. She gives me a solo, enthusiastic standing ovation at the end of class. I see her in the parking lot, guiding a toddler toward the car. This time for herself was temporary, celebrated.

Ellen lets go, forgetting her body's inhibitions.

Katie is steady.

Tracey is sassy.

Brooke is centered.

Emily puts everything on the floor when she dances. He joy and beauty fill the room. She loves to dance.

Surrounded by women I know; most are nameless. But we are here together often. We share energy and love, awareness and anonymity, complaints and praise. Community.

Some rush for the front row. Others hide in the back. Some complain — about anything, everything. Some complaints are serious while most are the usual search for camaraderie or attention. Some of us take our workouts seriously. Some just show up and zone out. We breathe passion. Some light up the room; others shrug off their shadows.

They say thank you. We love your classes. I am humbled.

Questions, comments, concerns, requests?

Faces and bodies fade and recombine. She's been here every time. I forgot her name, or forgot to ask. We've talked several times. She reminds me of someone. I hope she comes back....

Bodies on Edge

we feel it
the rise, the beat —
uncontainable.
in the car, at the store, on the couch
it moves us

we shake: anticipation

we feel it
the rise, the beat —
uncontrollable.
inside/outside (beyond reach)
it moves us

we shake: exhilaration

we are bodies on edge;
we are ripe craving movement

sharing space,
our bodies vibrate as one
rising, beating
shaking

          a groove
          a moment
          a lifetime

we feel it
the rise, the beat —

Fitness and Sexuality: Over and Under

If aerobics is often found by researchers to be disempowering, and if part of this has to do with the sexualized movements, then perhaps this says more about how sex and sexiness are seen in our culture than it does about the assumed disempowerment of the movements themselves. Fit bodies are over-sexualized from athletes to models; and non-white bodies are made more sexual as they are exoticized. Being more sexy, more appealing, and more attractive to the opposite (or same) sex, are often goals of exercise. Sexual appeal and attraction are also commonly understood as "biology" or evolution-based human nature; however, sexuality is different from manufactured ideas about sex appeal or beauty and fitness. A better sex life is an often-recognized benefit of fitness, cited not only by women's fashion and fitness magazines, but also by scientific studies, and in relation to all kinds of fitness programs from yoga to cardio striptease. Sex and sexuality are present on every glistening surface and yet also just out of sight. This is not one of those benefits that fitness instructors remind us of as we are shaking our hips or thrusting our pelvis. The average exerciser might recognize the sexy nature of moves but she might not know that the hype behind the exercise and sex connection is not simply hype. Regardless, sex is often a confused subject in the realm of fitness.

Sex and sexuality are recognized in relation to fitness even as they are pushed to the edges, smoothed out in euphemism and vague reference, or in service of patriarchal expectations. Some of the more taboo edges of sexuality are mentioned in Broad's exploration of the science of yoga. For instance, his chapter on "Divine Sex" is explained as a kind of after-thought, something he didn't really plan on writing but then just couldn't stay away from. People certainly make connections that cannot be ignored like Hot Nude Yoga classes, for instance.[8] While Broad focuses somewhat on tantric yoga, which is known for its sexual powers, his chapter turns to scientific knowledge that has been explored in places such as the documentary-style show, *Strange Sex*, which highlights unusual sexual interests and abilities. Both Broad and the Learning Channel's TV show, *Strange Sex,* feature women like Barbara Carrellas who can "think themselves off," who can orgasm without being touched and without touching themselves. Carrellas founded Urban Tantra "as a way of bringing people together to explore the vast range of sexual, spiritual and emotional possibilities open to all of us." While Broad is skeptical of many of yoga's other claims, this ability to orgasm using strictly the mind has been proven through scientific studies. But this science of yoga, while certainly a draw for some, is also uncomfortable for others who might steer clear of yoga for the fear of tapping into its sexual powers. Broad doesn't seem to notice the ways in which he veers away from the subject of yoga; he is still firmly in mind/body territory. Ultimately, such studies speak more to the power of the brain than to the power of fitness, but they are not far-fetched from the mysteries and pleasures of the mind/body connection.

Besides, yoga is regularly associated with sex, as the previously mentioned "Yoga Girl" video spoofs and as the 2003 film *Hollywood Homicide* illustrates through its rookie cop character, Kasey Calden, portrayed by Josh Hartnett.

As a wanna-be actor, Calden takes up teaching yoga; he admits to Harrison Ford's character (as waves of beautiful women thank him for class) that at first his teaching was for the sex, but then he found the spiritual aspects and he can't live without it. Yoga plays an odd role in this film, but its connections with sexuality are key to the character of this heart-throb cop. Another film example comes from the 2009 *Couples Retreat* where the tanned, muscled guru leads couples yoga. He not only puts the couples into suggestive positions, he also puts himself into these positions (awkwardly) as he "transfers energy" and flirts with the wives, particularly Lucy (Kristin Davis of *Sexy and the City* fame). Since sex is ultimately what fixes (or reinforces) the couple's relationships, perhaps this yoga element is fitting. The stories of sex and yoga have many variations.

The documentary, *Yoga, Inc.*, questions the poignancy of yoga as it points out that Rodney Yee, who once proclaimed yoga to be the foundation of his marriage left his family for a fellow yoga instructor. A 2005 article by Abigail Pogrebin, "An Illicit Yoga Love Story," explains some of the details of this affair as well as the controversies surrounding it and the subtitle sets the tone: "when the 'stud-muffin guru' hooked up with his student, disciples were left reeling." While Yee — a celebrated and popular yogi — touted yoga as the "backbone" of his marriage, he left his wife and children for a woman (Colleen Saidman) who left her husband of 24-years. Pogrebin notes, "despite their apparent fulfillment, Saidman concedes they're not poster children for proper conduct on the mat: 'The teacher-student relationship is very complicated. That can definitely be taken advantage of by a teacher. And I think a teacher shouldn't go there. Even though we did.'" This hypocritical message does not sit well with many yoga students, as the comments on this online article attest. Perhaps because he is seen as the "stud-muffin guru" and Saidman is less well-known, Yee takes the brunt of the criticism.

Such sexualized and sensationalized aspects of fitness also lead to the kinds of connections that discredit fitness and women generally, and specialized forms of dance fitness more specifically. Aerobics generally, and forms of aerobics like cardio belly dancing or Strip Tease Aerobics or Flirty Girl Fitness, specifically, make overt connections between sexiness and fitness. In "Keep Your Clothes On! Fit and Sexy Through Striptease Aerobics" Magdalena Petersson McIntyre explains a similar trend to "Flirty Girl Fitness" that appeared in Swedish health clubs in 2007 — Striptease aerobics. Like "Flirty Girl Fitness" this form of aerobics depends upon sexualized movements and assumptions about femininity, even as there is room for different kinds of expressions and negotiations of meanings, as McIntyre illustrates. What is interesting here, though, is that the media coverage made direct connections between the U.S. and Hollywood in its headlines and stories about the trend.

McIntyre notes that the inspiration came from "New York fitness trends and exercise videos sold on the Internet by Hollywood celebrity Carmen Electra" (249). And the headlines noted that the trend was "finally" available in Sweden. Thus, the American aspects of fitness are easily relatable in other westernized fitness contexts and, in this case, constitute a selling point for potential clients and an item of interest for the general public.

Zumba is also closely associated with sexiness; through its non-verbal emphasis, for instance, the focus is on the instructor's body. Her (or his) body speaks the cues and movements and provides the motivation. And many of the moves — like almost all dance moves — involve shaking the hips and hopping and moving in ways that could be seen as "suggestive." The suggestive nature of dance fitness forms then become attached to sex scandals like the 2012 scandal in Kennebunk, Maine. After unusual foot traffic revealed suspicious activity at her Pura Vida studio, Alexis Wright, a 29-year-old Zumba instructor, was arrested and charged with over 109 counts of prostitution, tax evasion, invasion of privacy and other charges. Her alleged accomplice, a 57-year-old insurance agent and private investigator, was charged with 59 misdemeanors. This controversy unfolded first in local news and then made national news headlines when the courts began considering releasing the names of the men charged with "engaging in prostitution" and several of the names included Maine's elite businessmen and politicians. The connection with a Zumba instructor added to the interest level of this prostitution story. It gives fuel to the stereotypes, seethes with controversy, and brings attention to this more affluent area of Maine. Women — as an extension of this woman — are implicated as pawns in the large scheme of fitness and patriarchal sexuality.

Wright plead guilty to 20 counts of prostitution, and at her sentencing hearing, Wright made a nine-minute statement that was posted online (almost instantly). On the NBC News website (via U.S. News) the headline read: "Zumba instructor sentenced to 10 months in jail on prostitution charges." A few pieces of her statement are mentioned, including her "traumatic childhood in which she was the victim of sexual abuse" (Arkin), as the story quotes Wright's lawyer. What is not contextualized for us are the parts of Wright's statement when she refers to being manipulated and forced to do things she did not want to do, to be a person she did not want to be. She expresses her relief and joy at the fact that this part of her life (which lasted and escalated over 10 years) was finally over. She speaks out to other women who are still in similar situations and vows to work with such women after she is released from jail. (A part that is included in the story.) She states that she had wanted to tell someone what was happening to her, but that she never thought they would believe her. She thanks her network of family and friends, including her husband who has stood by her, and looks forward to moving on with her life. Her alleged business partner received a 20-day sentence and a $3000 fine; his sentence was reduced by five days for good behavior. The story told in her statement to the judge is quite different than the story told in the blurbs about this prostitution scandal that "rocked" a small town in Maine. The punishments decreed by law, in light of this story, speak directly to the problems of patriarchy, capitalism, and sexism. The sexy Zumba instructor bears the brunt of the guilt, punished through direct and indirect impacts — the ramifications of legal and media institutions at work.

* * *

Ultimately, sex and sexuality are important parts of a balanced life and an improved sex life — for body and mind — is one of the many benefits of fitness. The schizophrenic and superficial ideas about sex in our American culture lead to disconnection and skewed expectations and practices. Fitness at the edges blurs sex, sexuality, and many variations of love.

Loving Women (Loving Self) Through Fitness

"Fitness was not a thing back then [1973]; *aerobics* was barely a word. Girls were supposed to be soft, and only the girls we suspected were butch could climb the ropes at school."
— Alice Sebold, *The Lovely Bones* (12)

"Consciously choosing to be a life force inside of love's ecosystem is a way to actually thrive. It requires imagination, a sense of humor, creativity, resourcefulness, openheartedness, and figuring out how to make the very, very best out of the very, very worst."
— Inga Muscio, *Rose: Love in Violent Times* (261)[9]

So many of us come to fitness for any and every reason; so many of us stay because we love it. But our understanding of love is incomplete and rarely articulated in its full complexity. Our love for ourselves might be buried beneath inhibitions or flaunted selfishly; our love for fitness shines through smiles as well as groans. But our love for each other is more difficult to express outside the confines of concerns with physical ailments or signed cards for an assortment of occasions — joyful to mournful. This contained expression is, in part, a result of our culture's reigns on love. Sexiness can be negotiated and flaunted, but sexuality is less visible or assumed to be irrelevant to the work(out).

There are many ways of loving women through fitness — love is a fundamental concept of feminist fitness — self-love and unconditional love for others. Because of the continuing (but slowly changing) stigma surrounding homosexuality, this love is never/rarely described as *lesbian*. As fitness reinforces the perfect body and narrow ideas of femininity, it also reinforces compulsory heterosexuality. We must be working out to look good for men; and the music and banter often reinforce this. For instance, when a song refers to a female love interest, the song will be performed by a male and when the song refers to a male love interest, the performer will be female. And if the love interest does not fit with, for instance, the heterosexual female instructor's personal interest, she might change the song as she instructs. For instance, in one song we met a group of girls in a particular car, and one instructor changed the girls in the car to a bunch of cute guys as she was cueing. When we danced to "Hot Girls" she explicitly mentioned that we need some "hot guys." So, while heterosexuality is already assumed, it is reinforced through such manipulations. Are we afraid we might be seen as gay if we play along with the music?[10]

Many feminists describe the ways in which the lesbian label is used to "bait" women, to undercut a woman who has power or influence. Suzanne Pharr explains that a woman is considered a lesbian any time she challenges patriarchal expectations. She explains, "the word lesbian is instilled with power to halt our work and control our lives. And we give it power with our fear" (74). The word, Lesbian, like the word Feminist, has the ability to disempower, but lesbian does so even more powerfully because lesbian sexuality is the ultimate slap in the face of patriarchy. So are strong women at the gym. But lesbians are a diverse group of women, defined differently in terms of sexuality. Just like any other women, Pharr explains some lesbians are:

> in long-term relationships, some in short-term ones, some date, some are celibate, some are married to men, some remain as separate as possible from men, some have children by men, some by alternative insemination, some seem "feminine" by societal standards, some "masculine," some are doctors, lawyers and ministers, some laborers, housewives and writers: what all share in common is a sexual/affectional identity that focuses on women in its attractions and social relationships [73].

In short, lesbian women are diverse and do not fall into easy categories or stereotypes. And if "attractions" and "social relationships" define fitness spaces as well as lesbian consciousness, recognition and development of individual and collective lesbian identity is the missing component in fitness. In fitness, lesbian identity is wrapped up in stereotypes about fit women — the "butch" girls who could "climb the rope in school." Lesbian consciousness is not a comfortable term for the love that women share in the studio, even if the idea and practice are reality.

* * *

In fitness spaces, social coding of compulsory heterosexuality reigns. Despite the presence of lesbian women in the celebrity world of fitness — for instance, Jillian Michaels (of *The Biggest Loser* fame) and Jackie Warner — the gym continues to be a hostile space for many kinds of otherness, including gays and lesbians.[11] However, there are also feminist fitness personalities that seek to interrupt not only the heteronormativity of fitness but also the ways in which mainstream fitness approaches skew the true meaning of fitness.

In a 2004 *Curves* magazine article, Susan Powter described herself as a "radical, feminist, lesbian woman." Powter had a short-lived TV show, *The Susan Powter Show*, in 1994 and has been a best-selling *NY Times* author three times. She gained fitness fame from her infomercials, aired during the early 90s. She was instantly recognizable by her short-cropped bleached-blond hair and her forceful voice and personality. As a montage of diet claims fills the screen, Susan yells, "Stop the Insanity!" In her infomercials she uses her personal weight loss of 133 pounds as a means to motivate other women to do what she did. And her first line after her famous catch phrase is, "diets don't work." She tells her audience that she didn't go from being a fat person to a thin person over night. In fact, she says, "I went from an unfit person to a fit person." She does not promote thinness, but the ability to climb stairs without getting winded.

In her blog titled "making edible playdough is hegemonic: notes toward resistance," Jenna McWilliams includes a post: "Susan Powter Is a Lesbian." In this blog she reminds us of who Powter is/was and states "she's a big old dyke now." (This is a compliment. As McWilliams also states, "We need all the radical feminist lesbian women we can get.") Being married twice and having three kids (one adopted) was a good disguise for Powter as she was able to reach out to her audience through heterosexual commonality. For instance, in her infomercial she says "ask my ex-husband...." and describes her credentials not as a doctor or a nutritionist but as "a house wife that figured it out." And yet, on AfterEllen.com, a 2008 article proclaims, "Susan Powter thinks it should be obvious she's a lesbian." This post comments on her appearance on *The Morning Show with Mike and Juliet* where they try to "confront her" about being a lesbian. She confirms the fact, even asking, "What planet were you on?" and moves them back to the subject at hand.

More recently, Susan Powter has reappeared with her website, which claims, "the insanity stops here," and her "Eat, Breathe, Move, Think" approach to fitness. A variety of services are available on Powter's website and she makes short video blogs that might affectionately be called rants — commentary from Susan Powter on a variety of fitness-related subjects. Powter's somewhat abrasive personality comes through; she is outspoken and opinionated and raw. In the middle of several rants she asks, "Do I have crap in my teeth again?" and "Look at my hair." She calls attention to her appearance and yet urges her viewers to focus on other fitness qualities.

Susan critiques and responds to a variety of pop culture figures and trends including Richard Simmons as she threatens to kick his ass for calling her an "evil harpy." Powter's somewhat nonsensical no nonsense approach cuts right through the crap that the media spews over and over. She calls to task women like Rachel Ray who help to perpetuate myths and misunderstandings related to fitness (like convenience and "reducing weight to some emotion"), but speaks to the bigger picture. Fitness is "bigger than" the anecdotes and the before and after pictures; as Powter notes, if not in these words, the American lifestyle of convenience and non-reflection are not conducive to realistic fitness goals.

While some might be intimidated by her personality, or even her sexuality, Powter continues to do the work that is important to her — promoting a common sense kind of approach to weight loss and motivating women to find a real, connected relationship with their bodies through their minds. Sometimes she veers toward the superficial, but always couched in radical feminism that holds the system accountable and asks us to be conscious of the manipulations of mainstream fitness ideas.

* * *

"In order to unlearn monogamy and liberate our sexuality, we need to uproot the arbitrary limitations to our thinking and seeing that have been imposed on our minds by previous philosophies.... Sluthood can become a path to transcendence, a freeing of the mind and spirit as well as the body, a way of being in the world that allows expanded awareness, spiritual growth, and — not incidentally — really good sex."
— *The Ethical Slut: A Guide to Infinite Sexual Possibilities* (266–7)

It was through fitness and through academic theory, that I realized my bisexuality, that I am physically and mentally attracted to women. Despite the fact of my marriage to a man, I spend most of my time with women. Most of my work is about women and toward the benefit of women. Most of the people I work with on a regular basis are women. Most of the people I work with — as colleagues and participants in the world of fitness — are women. Most of my friends are women and many of them are out lesbians. And, yet, I rarely come out. Sometimes I follow the lead of Alison Bechdel's character Sparrow, who describes herself as a Bisexual Lesbian Feminist. But most of the time this is not the kind of confession, or celebration, that is worked into a class between the cardio portion and the final stretch or during final relaxation. In and out of the gym, it is really just too much to explain, and not really anyone's business. The women I love in fitness stay at the level of friends — a result of professional distance, a lack of confidence in my romantic/sexual appeal to women, and a result of a heart broken by a fitness crush that bloomed into love. I was only beginning to discover the many forms of love, to challenge the "arbitrary limitations."

Long before I was aware of what I felt for Erin, I would idolize her as a participant in the same step class I took — a credit step aerobics class. I would hide in the middle of the room. She was always up front. She clearly idolized the teacher and she would approach her own workout holding nothing back — sweating and grunting and squeaking out encouragement for the instructor's work. She took the class with a friend and they were always there to set up their steps early. I would watch her avarice; she rarely, if ever, missed a step. She was passionate about the same kinds of things I was passionate about. But I only ever watched her from a distance.

Later we worked together at the fitness center on campus and she took the fitness instructor training course that I helped to teach. Eventually we became friends, in part because of our love of fitness classes, our interest in choreography, and our similar philosophical and political interests outside the fitness studio. We were both "would-be world savers" like two of Octavia Butler's characters in her *Parables* series.[12] Only later, I would learn how different our politics really were. For some time, fitness kept us bonded and fostered other kinds of bonds between us.

Our friendship developed into something more. She made me feel free to express myself and I would write her love letters, and intellectually-driven e-mails where we would debate bisexuality and she would share her sexual exploits with men (of which there were many). I would profess my love and she would tell me of her latest crush. I bought her a book I discovered — *The Ethical Slut* — as I pursued ways of explaining my ideas about love and sex and sexuality. I thought love could be simple, multiple, and boundless. She was my best friend (though, as is the pattern of most of my friendships, she had another friend who was technically her best friend) and she was one of the few friends my husband and I both got along with. I was 24, the age I had dreamed about as a girl, the age when I thought I would be an adult and I would know everything and I would have everything together. As a child I could see myself at age 24 because I could imagine the year 2000, a time that seemed so impossibly far away. I never saw beyond the year 2000 as I would speculate what my age would be at designated points in the future. Thus, at 24 the world seemed endlessly possible and I thought I had the power to make the world, or at least my world, what I wanted it to be.

I would take her classes — most often step classes. I would enjoy the steps and the choreography and the music and the experience of fitness and have the added pleasure of watching her body move. For a short time she also taught yoga and my husband and I would be the only one who attended. On the third floor with a skylight and just the three of us, yoga felt magical, serene, perfect. We would practice together and she taught me ways to develop my kickboxing combos into more complex and interesting sets of moves, ways to travel and change directions. We would critique other instructors and we would bike, rock climb, play softball, and hike together as well. We went to the farmer's market and shared many vegetarian meals. She first peaked my interest in a vegan diet though I could not give up my love of cheese. I loved her unconditionally.

But our closeness did not last and other things got in the way: her obvious attraction to other women instead of me, her endless crushes on any man that gave her a second look, my insecurity and lack of comfort pursuing this new interest in my life, jealousies of other friends, my romanticized vision of her and of how to make polyamory work, the awkward sex that was all about her. She blamed my insecurity. I blamed her selfishness. But ultimately I blamed myself for my lack of balance. I let her be everything and that is too much to expect from anyone. Loving Erin was an exercise in loving self. I had to learn to love myself and I had to learn to not let love fester.

I left town to pursue my Ph.D., but we had stopped talking before then. Through fitness, though not exclusively, I had opened the door to a world of possibility. Subconsciously, deliberately, submissively, I seemed to close the door on the possibility of boundless love. I lost a part of myself that was, perhaps, replaced by a more mature, and much less bold, version of the old. And yet the love is there, under the surface, pushed to the corners. Self-love, and love for other women, pulses inside of me and is expressed, in part, through my love for fitness. The non-threatening space where loving women can be both visible and masked feeds my soul. I sometimes develop mostly platonic crushes on fitness instructors. These are crushes of admiration and a kind of envy, a desire to be them (and still, somehow, myself) and a settling to just be *with* them. I enjoy watching women in fitness classes, watching the ways their bodies move, watching their concentration and enjoyment. This is a pleasure I allow myself to only partially embrace, and, yet, fitness will certainly yield many more versions of love over time. It is a space of possibility.

* * *

Feminist writers like Inga Muscio and feminist critics like bell hooks and Chela Sandoval, write about love. Like "fitness," the concept of love is complex, narrowly represented in pop culture, and understood through limited experience. Sandoval and hooks, and critics like Paulo Freire, also explore a pedagogy of love. This pedagogy informs my teaching in academia and in fitness. Too few people in academia are brave enough to speak about love as a pedagogy[13] — as bell hooks argues, the love we have for our subject matter is a far more comfortable kind of love (particularly for administrators) than the love we have for our students. The love we have for our students is seen as a problem, a hindrance to our objectivity and an emotional state that impedes our work in the classroom. But bell hooks also makes a case for love as an important part of critical, feminist pedagogy, a way of enhancing students' classroom experiences, individually and in community. Love, hooks argues, is "a combination of care, commitment, knowledge, responsibility, respect, and trust. All these factors work interdependently. They are a core foundation of love irrespective of the relational context" (131). In writing about "love in violent times" Inga Muscio argues that love "requires imagination, a sense of humor, creativity, resourcefulness, openheartedness, and figuring out how to make the very, very best out of the very, very worst" (261). Ultimately, our discomfort with the subject of love and pedagogy is an extension of, and function of, our larger problems with understanding and defining love in a culture where one word is expected to represent all of the various inflections, dimensions, and shades of "love." As bell hooks continues, "Even though there is a difference between romantic love and the love between teacher and pupil, these core aspects must be present for love to be love" (131).

I love my students. Throughout my education this loving pedagogy didn't really take a concrete shape in my mind, or a decisive name. I found such pedagogy largely through intuition, application, reflection, and, when more formally recognized, through Paulo Freire and bell hooks' writings.[14] Mostly I just taught based upon intuition and the critical consciousness I was developing through my education. In the various contexts where I learned to teach, pedagogy was not the priority. So, formal instruction in pedagogy was largely absent and, like I did for most of my education, I have continued to piece together something that would work for me. It is only recently that I have come to understand that love, as both bell hooks and Inga Muscio define it above, is the best way to describe my pedagogy. The editors of *Feminist Pedagogy* explain:

> Feminist teachers demonstrate sincere concern for their students as people and as learners and communicate this care through treating students as individuals, helping students make connections between their studies and their personal lives, and guiding students through the process of personal growth that accompanies their intellectual development [5].

I care for and commit to my students. I trust them and respect them and share knowledge and responsibility in collaborative relationships with students, in and out of the classroom. I work to help students make important connections and to see that personal growth is often part and parcel with learning. "Imagination, a sense of humor, creativity, resourcefulness, [and] openheartedness" describe the ways in which I approach the difficult subject matter I teach through American studies and women's studies — from identity, culture, and politics to racism, white supremacy, and patriarchy to consciousness, community, and transformation.

There is also risk in a loving pedagogy as we open ourselves to the possibility of what bell hooks describes as mutuality; we must be conscious as teachers. We must recognize the importance of "boundaries" — one of my biggest struggles. After learning that such a concept even exists, I have skirted the edges as I continue to give too much. Boundaries, I have recently learned — aren't simply about keeping others out; they're about keeping our own self from spilling or seeping out. One of my reasons for a lack of boundaries is an inability to say no when I think other people need me; even the need for self-preservation makes it difficult to stop giving. So I keep moving, working it out; students are inevitably a part of this process. As bell hooks argues, "between teacher and student love makes recognition possible; it offers a place where the intersection of academic striving meets the overall striving to be psychologically whole" (136). Such an intersection requires us to be fully present for our students and uneven, power-laden collaboration can undercut love: "the conditions for optimal learning" (136). Like academic engagement, psychological wholeness is not something to be broken down and rebuilt from the fragments of self, it is something to be fostered, bolstered, enhanced, and transformed. Critical consciousness, feminist pedagogy, and a pedagogy of love makes such wholeness possible for students *and* teachers. "Psychological wholeness" can be found in the fitness studio as love combats the power of "fat" to define and confine.

Feminism Makes You Fat

"I expect a certain amount of fat bias in every [fitness] class I attend. After all, the majority of the country has the (scientifically false) idea that fatness and fitness are mutually exclusive. And I'm under no illusions. I know that many people take fitness classes just so *they won't end up looking like me.* Sigh."
— Tiffany Kell, "Project Bendypants: Practicing Yoga While Fat"

A by-product of the "perfect body" means that "fat" is the enemy — to be purged via fitness if not more drastic means. Since women are so caught up in body image — a direct confluence with media representations and patriarchal expectations — one sure-fire way to discredit feminism is to link it with the dreaded specter of "fat." Despite increases in "women's sports and exercise participation," we still have not excised the "cosmetic" aspect of fitness.[15] We might even assume this increased participation is because of a desire to meet the ever-stricter guidelines of superficiality. The inclusion of an entire section in *Women and Exercise* devoted to "Body Trouble: Fat Women and Exercise" means that concerns about fatness continue to circulate as powerful motivators and determents of fitness for women.

In "Large Women's Experiences of Exercise" the authors (Groven, et al.) discuss the fact that they use the term "large" instead of "fat" or obese because it is "less stigmatizing" (121). Regardless of how it is phrased, "fat" continues to be a concern of women because it is a bigger concern of our appearance-obsessed culture. As Louise Mansfield argues in "Fit, Fat and Feminine? The Stigmatization of Fat Women in Fitness Gyms," while fat was never on her research agenda, the topic could not be avoided since fat became a key subject in all of her discussions with women. Women's perceptions of their bodies "were oriented toward ideas about fat.... All those I spoke with defined themselves in relation to fat; losing fat, gaining fat, being and becoming fat, and fearing fat" (84). The large women studied by Groven, et al. wanted to lose weight not for the sake of health but "normalcy" (134). Thus, body size is both a powerful draw and stumbling block when it comes to pursuits of fitness. The norm of fat is stigmatized as not "normal," while the pictures we see in the media are anything but normal. Brabazon discusses the ways in which "fat" is posed as a "problem" to be dealt with through counseling. (73) Feminism has yet to break the cultural power of the fear of fat. In fact, ideas like "feminism makes you fat" clog up our understanding.

In her 2010 blog post, Lisa Johnson, of the website Lisa Johnson Fitness, "everything for a healthy body" opens with the title, "Feminism Makes You Fat." She writes, "a rather provocative headline, isn't it? Yet, there is a little ripple going around foodie circles right now that believes just that. Let me state these are progressive, liberal people making this claim. And they actually have a bit of a point." She is referring to a statement made by foodie, Michael Pollan in *The New York Review of Books*.[16] She goes on to explain:

> Basically, the more that women work out of the home, the less likely we are to cook healthy meals for our family. Stop. Breathe. Think about it for a second. This seems a little plausible, doesn't it? ... I try to cook meals at home as much as I can. It's really important to me that my family eat well.... But when life gets busy, I'm reaching for the take out menu just like everyone else.

The argument is, as Johnson explains, an important one to consider. The *ways* in which we eat, and the *things* we eat, have been greatly impacted by cultural changes — a wide spectrum of cultural changes that are not simply the result of feminism. For instance, global economic trends and American policies are responsible for women having to work outside the home even if feminism made women's "choice" to work a part of its agenda (and for many women, particularly, women of color, such choice was never a choice in the first place). The assumption that women should be able to work and still produce healthy meals for their families is a powerful cultural message, even if it is unstated. Further, the abundance of unhealthy meal choices have been manufactured to fill this socio-cultural void, and profits (not health) are the concern and creation of business men.

Feminism — an ideal that opposes the injustices associated with these cultural changes — is the easy scapegoat. When an anti-feminist takes up the topic, the conversation is posed in quite a different way. As Kevin Smith Game argues in his 2012 blog post, "Feminism is Making America Fat." By encouraging women to enter the workforce, feminism also encouraged women to "leave the homeforce in droves." The result is, as Johnson notes as well, fewer home-cooked meals and more trips through the take-out window. Game's evidence is not much different from Johnson's, even if his delivery and conclusions are quite opposite. The difference are most clear when he writes about his solution:

> You want to reframe the national discourse so that feminism is killed dead before it has a chance to infect the next generation of hosts? Just tell a woman about to embark on a contorted feminist line of reasoning that feminism makes people fat. If you want to win hearts and minds, you've gotta hit 'em where it matters. And for women, it matters most in the size of their figures.

It seems that Game is less concerned about the realities of "the American obesity epidemic" and more concerned with using this as an opportunity to "reframe the national discourse so that feminism is killed dead before it has a chance to infect the next generation of hosts." And yet, his demeaning assumption that telling a woman that "feminism makes people fat" will make her drop her feminist interests is absurd and insulting to women's intelligence even as it holds a kernel of truth: women *are* concerned with their size. Is this concern a powerful form of kryptonite to feminists everywhere? It doesn't have to be.

Game's assumptions are searing judgments of women's concerns about "the size of their figures." Of course, his analysis does not hint that this concern is conditioned by a culture shaped by men like him. His sentiments here are a more insidious form of Kenneth Cooper's "findings" regarding women. More than 40 years later we might wonder at the impact of feminism. Clearly Game's argument is reactionary, simplistic, inflammatory and incomplete, but his post, filed under "feminist idiocy," resulted in more than 350 comments while Johnson's post only garnered twelve, many of which are her own replies to others' comments.[17] While Game's post is an opportunity to bash the "contorted feminist line of reasoning," Johnson's is a conversation that seeks to change a damaging cultural message about women, for women.

* * *

In "Fit, Fat and Feminine? The Stigmatization of Fat Women in Fitness Gyms" Louise Mansfield argues that "gyms are a place where fears and anxieties about fat are mobilized" (85). And, obviously, her research illustrates this fact. However, there are many cultural spaces where "fears and anxieties about fat are mobilized." These are deeply entrenched cultural beliefs and our anxieties are played out in entertainment as well as advertising for reinforcement. Women who are considered obese, fat, overweight, large, chunky, thick, big-boned, or flabby stand out in fitness environments that have the "perfect body" as their goal and idealized picture of health and fitness. Women who are older are seen as frail, a nuisance. However, at the gym, outside of the gym, and through all kinds of fitness, women of a certain age and a certain weight can feel welcome, whole, and energized. This work might be one of the most difficult interventions in mainstream fitness. In "Growing Old (Dis)Gracefully? The Gender/Aging/Exercise Nexus," Elizabeth C. J. Pike contextualizes the exercise of older women within a culture that devalues aging women, in part because of the growing numbers of the world's population over 60 years old, of which women comprise a majority. She refers to "'the age of aging'" and the social anxieties that surround aging, including the framing of "longer life expectancy" as "a problem" in terms of "impact on the economy, social and health care services, and even the environment" (180–1). These preconceived notions mean that the public might see the health and fitness of older Americans as unimportant, even as the ironies abound.

Separately, the dominant fitness ideas of youthfulness and thinness might be discouraging, but together they can become nearly impenetrable. Further, the expectations that go along with these ideals are also discouraging, or even damaging to older and larger women exercisers. For instance the idea that exercise is serious work, coupled with culturally valuable ideas of "no pain no gain" and "not giving up" (Groven, et al. 126), have contributed to negative experiences in relation to exercise for larger women. In fact, "'pushing oneself' was interpreted as a culturally positive value" (Groven, et al. 131) even when this value was in direct conflict with the discomfort, boredom, or even pain of the experience. These myths circulate widely amongst exercisers of many shapes and sizes, ages and approaches, but they are most dangerous for those of us who have special fitness concerns like injuries, medical conditions, or other factors, like body size and age, that deserve an individualized approach without stigmatization.

While some of the large women studied by Groven, et al. had experienced positive exercise forms outside of the circuit training module of their study, for the most part these women did not associate exercise with pleasure or enjoyment. Instead, "pleasure was regarded as a reward *after* exercising" (130). The authors argue that programs that are painful and not fun "can result in the participants' constant dissatisfaction and ill health" (136). Thus, "success measured through the reduction of body size is problematic" (135). For large women such results are not necessarily achievable, despite what weight loss narratives might promote. And for older women, results must be seen outside of the context of the "perfect body" as a youthful body since this too is an impossible standard. The purpose of exercise must be different from these desired results as well.

* * *

Perhaps one of the most recognizable fitness personalities around, Richard Simmons has made a name for himself "Sweatin' to the Oldies" and supporting marginalized exercisers (the older, larger, and poorer), and he is still going strong. With 50 DVDs, nine books, three cookbooks, he offers a wealth of fitness-related information, mostly to those at the margins of the fitness world. He speaks from his heart about his struggles with obesity and how he turned his life around. He opened his studio, SLIMMONS, in Beverly Hills in the early 1970s as a "safe haven" for "any and every one." He does not shirk from the overweight who comprise a large portion of his audience. And he reaches out to an older American audience with other programs like "Sit Tight," a workout for those who can't stand up when they work out. More than anything, Simmons is a motivator; for instance, he also has a DVD, "Love Yourself and Win" and "Straight from the Heart: Richard's Secrets to Success." In Los Angeles in 2004 he began "Hoot Camp." According to his bio: "this is a grassroots effort that Richard will take to outreaching communities where he teaches fitness teachers and coaches how to motivate their students by incorporating humor and persona into their classes." Richard has even jumped on the latest fitness bandwagon, offering his own version of the 90-day weight loss program, Project H.O.P.E." Richard's energy is, we might hope, infectious. His bio looks forward rather than spending its time looking back on his hay day. "Remembering his childhood as an obese kid and prime target of neighborhood bullies, Richard also plans to embark on an educational program for children and their parents in the New Year, reaching this under-represented population before their fitness fate is sealed." He continues to dream big. Despite his fame, Richard occupies the edges of fitness.

While Richard Simmons' fitness brand is motivational, we might also consider the ways in which we are able to subvert (and maybe even transform) the cultural expectations of young and thin as measures of healthy and fit. Tiffany Kell's "Project Bendypants" (and the Decolonizing Yoga website, more generally) challenge dominant perceptions of "fat" as well as the "principles of compassion and reflection that yoga is built around." Despite her physical/athletic abilities in other fitness classes, Kell struggles with flexibility and this struggle — one of her reasons for attending class — adds to many yoga teachers' superficial judgments. She writes, "I apparently committed an unspoken offense to many of the yoga teachers I encountered: I attempted to practice yoga while fat." Kell's "crime" is the exact thing that so many of us fear; it keeps us away from the gym.

While there is all of this concern over fighting fat, organizations like National Association to Advance Fat Acceptance (NAAFA) "have demonstrated ... that the fat body can be a fit body" (73). Brabazon mentions the story of Kathryn Szrodecki who qualified to be an aerobics instructor weighing 200 pounds. Szrodecki critiques the industry that tells women that they can be a certain size if they just try hard enough. She writes, "'This is a lie'" (as quoted by Brabazon, 73). She speaks a truth vigilantly battled by famous fitness personalities like the previously-mentioned, Susan Powter. As Brabazon notes, "a strong, fit, big woman is a powerful symbol of what femininity can be, when stripped from the medicalised [sic] discourse" (74). I would easily fit into the "fat" category, and I know women participants and instructors who are also "fat" and yet fit as well. If "fat" can't identify for us the culprits of the "problems" associated with body mass, our measures and perceptions have to change.

Appreciation of the older/larger body might include mindful, mind/body, slow movement practices like yoga, Nia, or the Putkisto Method. Interestingly, Parviainen notes that "Putkisto constantly emphasizes that the MP keeps the body looking youthful, but unlike mere body shaping, the method is 'working inside out' to improve the entire self" (44). Thus, the method includes an appeal to the anxieties and desires of older women — the desire to look youthful (as impossible as this might be in actuality) — while also providing an alternative methodology, one that will inevitably be safer and more enjoyable.

After all, as Groven, et al. argue, "being under constant pressure can be counterproductive for obtaining good health" (133). While the pressures of life are obviously counterproductive, a fitness plan that doesn't fit the individual's needs, goals, and interests creates insurmountable pressures. This is particularly true for those most marginalized by mainstream America.

Some critics call for different expectations for large women (Mansfield); the goals of fitness can be pleasure rather than pain, health rather than reduction. Others argue that we should "give more attention to their personal experiences and abilities" (Groven, et al. 135); the activities that we program for "certain" ages or body sizes might not be the best ones. There are many ways to be active, not all of which fit into "fitness" molds. Other critics argue that rather than relying upon current models for aging exercisers we should "enhance the celebration of life, experience, and character as it is written on the older woman's body and appreciate the beauty therein" (Pike 193). I try to sneak such moments into class. For instance, one Sunday my friend came to my Organic Dance class, and I made a special playlist for her birthday. I dedicated the class to the "joy of growing older." As the class was winding down and we finished stretching, I asked participants to reflect upon what joys they found in growing older. As Ani diFranco's "Not a Pretty Girl" faded out, I mentioned that we no longer had to be "pretty girls," that we could just be ourselves, and asked others to share their thoughts as we lay on our mats in "corpse" pose. I was almost surprised when I heard one voice after another sharing their own ideas, including freedom and empowerment. Their voices were strong.

Mind/body approaches to fitness embody many of the ideas of academic critics: different expectations, a focus on perception and experience, and celebration. For instance, Nia's idea of "The Body's Way," is an important mode for reconsidering the body. As Debbie and Carlos explain, "the Body's Way is a method of using the body in accord with its specific design and structure. It involves looking at the body as it really is, instead of viewing it in an idealized, conceptualized way" (30). The focus on how movement makes us feel rather than how exercise can make us look, is a more realistic approach and one that allows for the most honest assessments. The damaging messages of culture and its fear of fat are not able to poison perceptions of feeling. Likewise, Nia's "x-ray anatomy" (25, 72–4) takes the focus off of outer appearance and onto the structure of our bones, encouraging us to "see beneath [our] skin, using [our] eyes, intuition, and imagination" (73). These are powerful tools in and out of fitness — one tool that helps us see through limiting expectations.

Marja Putkisto, developed her method from a state of physical impairment. As Parviainen explains, Marja was urged by her doctor to give up the idea of a career in physical activity or fitness. But she refused to give up on this possibility and, instead, she continued to study dance and physical education. (47) Gabrielle Roth has a similar story, creating 5 Rhythms while recovering from an injury. Parviainen describes Pukisto's story as "heroic" and argues that this "heroic" aspect of the story, in addition to the movements of the program itself, "can be a powerful way for aging women to gain self-respect and gain their femininity" (56). Marja Putkisto is her own best example. As Parviainen argues, she "seems to be convinced that her own method has transformed her body and it offers a suitable tool to change others' bodies as well" (48). She is not wrong. While every body is different, if we remember to listen to our bodies and to integrate this knowledge with other sources — instructors and gurus, inventors and practitioners — we need not forget that our own bodies are an important starting point.

We navigate the edges — the limitations of our own bodies — a version of the nature versus nurture debates.

Mother Issues/Father Issues

> "Women of a certain age often become invisible to people ... as it is for most women going to the gym at any age, you have to be able to see yourself there before you can be comfortable there. I pay attention because I want to remember that this is possible."
> — Catherine Houser, "Enduring Images" (93)

While I remember my mother's pursuits toward fitness throughout my childhood, I also remember her during this time as a woman who was unhappy in her body. She was always on a diet (in words if not in practice); she was often trying a new fad. (We're both better at starting things than we are at finishing them.) But she also often did not have any time to focus on herself in addition to three kids with disparate schedules and a more-than-full-time job as a newspaper editor and reporter. And she was a product of the same kinds of antics her own mother would perform. Years after my grandmother died from ovarian cancer my mother shared with me a story about something she said on her deathbed. She said that she was finally the size she always wanted to be but that she now had nowhere to go. While my grandmother recognized that this thought and this statement were absurd, she had the thought and made the statement none-the-less. It was a truth. This ghost stays with the women of my family.

I remember my mother telling me about a girl she knew from school, a girl who was "flat-chested" and grew up to be the fitness superstar and workout tape diva, Kathy Smith. Sometimes my mother would muse about how it was easy for her to be thin; she was always skinny. Sometimes she would say something about the trade-off: she may be skinny but she doesn't have any boobs (a judgment that is clearly rooted in patriarchal expectations of beauty and a woman's value). Sometimes my mother would wonder why she could not be like Kathy Smith — they were the same age after all and came from the same place, more or less.

At the same time that my mother would talk about being unhappy with her body, or would be judging other women's bodies, or comparing herself to other women's bodies, feeling better or worse about her own body through the comparison, she would also assert herself as a feminist. Even though I did not know exactly what a feminist was — besides a woman who knew her rights — I knew, for sure, that my mother considered herself a feminist and that she and my father were raising me to have the idea that I could do anything and be anything that I wanted to be. But feminism was used as a negative: *No. You can't go see that new Andrew Dice Clay movie with all your friends. He degrades women.* And while the disconnect was not entirely conscious, there was doubt in my mind about the relationship between feminism and body politics. I would strive for an ideal body image without really knowing anything different. In my mind, the perfect body was equated with happiness, a contentment with self and body. An acceptance.

When fitness became something more than a way to pursue this body image, I began to transform my relationship between myself and my body, between the expectations that seemed to be embedded in my bones and brain and the meaning of fitness in my life and for my body. (But, the ghost remains.) And while my mother continues to make inane comments about the fat around her middle, or under her upper arms, and as she continues to consume beauty products with avarice, she has been transformed by a different approach to fitness — or perhaps by the realization that she does not have to be fat and unhappy. And exercise has made her happier with herself. She is more confident and more willing to be happy for herself.

My mother coached my soccer team when I was five years old, but I could never remember her doing anything physical like running or swimming or playing sports (unlike my father who played recreational softball and basketball). My mother, who spent many years of her life complaining about her body but not doing anything to change it, has become a biathlete. She has run and biked and walked many, many miles. She lifts weights with her personal trainer twice a week and takes yoga regularly. She even started teaching yoga and has done so regularly at her church and a local YMCA. A love of fitness is something we can share.

I might like to take some credit for this transformation. I'd like to think that after all of these years of her being my role model, I showed my mother the effects of fitness. After I began teaching yoga I convinced my mother to try a training, and she did. She began teaching yoga and she did other trainings (more than me!), and we were able to attend a YogaFit level three training together. We plan to take more trainings together though finding the time in our busy work schedules makes this difficult. I have relied upon my mother to get me through some of the "new-agey" aspects that every training includes, to be my accomplice in our critiques of the trainers. Like when, minutes after the yoga trainer had talked about the benefits of a vegetarian diet as a means to practice the yoga principle of ahimsa (non-violence), we broke for lunch; and when we volunteered to pick up lunch for her she asked for a salad — with as much meat as possible piled on top. What kind of meat did not matter, only the vastness of the quantity. We laughed, drank our smoothies, and complied with her wishes. Yoga has helped us to strengthen old bonds and to form new ones.

And so I see my mother transformed, and we both continue to struggle with that old ghost. Only recently did she confess to me that she has struggled with bulimia. We both binge. We cycle — gain and lose five, seven, ten, fifteen pounds. I binge but don't purge; I keep it all inside. I sit with my discomfort. These struggles are side effects of living a life in a culture that confines us to unrealistic expectations while also providing an abundance. These struggles are Feminism scratching at the edges of our worlds, moving us and expecting us to make the space. I find that the only way to survive, to maintain, is through movement. And movement leads to transformation ... however slow that transformation might be.

* * *

It would not be fair, or feminist, to complain of "mother issues" without also mentioning the related father issues. Mothers unfairly bear the brunt of issues and blame when it comes to the body. As Tara Brabazon argues, "It is convenient and appropriate in the midst of neo-conservatism not only to blame the individual food-disordered person for their 'problems' but also to share the blame with a dysfunctional mother" (77). Me, my mother, my father, my family and friends, all of us, are a part of this insidious system that requires that we blame ourselves for problems that originate in the culture-at-large.

Like my mother, my father was also always "fat" while I was growing up. When we finished our dinner he would clean all our plates; he came from a family where you didn't waste food. While my father did not excel at sports as a child, he loved them and as an adult he played softball and basketball recreationally and regularly coached me and/or my siblings. When he wasn't a coach, he was still an active supporter of our athletic events. They were, he hoped, a ticket to a college scholarship and, at the very least, they were developmentally important. Even though I cannot remember his presence at every game (he did have three kids' schedules to juggle, after all), I do remember him as a constant presence in my sporting life. He was always supportive of my mediocre athleticism. (My judgmental words, not his.)

My father's closest claims to sporting fame came from stories about his exploits as "belly bomping" champion, which seemed to me, as a child, a proud claim to fame rather than a lament. His beer belly was popularly known amongst our friends, and we knew that he had the nickname "Fat Ed." Not until much later in my life did I start to think that maybe these nicknames and this "fat" identity made him feel bad about himself. He never let on. But, of course, he was also raised on good old-fashioned masculinity. He was always what Michael Kimmel refers to as the "sturdy oak."[18] And he always emphasized the importance of brains; beauty or brawn weren't part of the equation.

I never connected my father's body issues with my own until I visited my parents well into adulthood. It was around Christmas time and my parents had received a tin of cookies from a friend or neighbor. As I shoved one in my mouth, something I never expected came out of my father's mouth. He said, "a moment on the lips a lifetime on the hips." I was shocked into silence. *Did that phrase really come out of my father's mouth?* I had never heard him say anything like that *ever*. I didn't think he paid attention to my body size and if he noticed, I didn't think he cared. Such conversations happened between me and my mother. I especially didn't expect him to turn to a worn-out adage. My father is far too smart and clever for that!

But this was a particular stage in my father's life when he lost weight — a lot of weight. My father's a kind of all-or-nothing type (and he passed this quality on to me) and so when he decided to lose weight he did so with gusto — with really, really long walks and with not a lot more food than beer and pretzels. This was not healthy weight loss, but it was effective. He went up and down with this until he had health problems. Since then, he has made a commitment to exercise and food that is a lot more healthy. Since retiring he has not only lost weight, but also regularly plays golf, walks, and bikes. He has even taken some yoga, to my shocked surprise. He keeps close count of his steps on his pedometer and gets in at least 30,000 steps a day. But, no doubt my father has his own food issues. So many of us do.

Both of my parents have inspired me. They've both committed to different forms of physical fitness and are happy and healthy in addition to being kind and generous people. In fact, as a result of timing, it was my father who inadvertently helped me practice better eating, to commit to having a different relationship with food, to stop struggling unproductively. Their struggles make them human. Perhaps my struggles make me more human as well. We share the same biology, but what we do with our natural resources is key to our fitness.

* * *

In my academic life, the power of social construction holds far more weight than any kind of biological, genetic determinism. And yet, the realities of genetic circumstances largely determine who and what we can become. LL Cool J notes that he is simply taking his "God-given genetics and mak[ing] the most out of them" (xii). He implies that these genetics are nothing special. Gina Kolata notes that in both aerobics conditioning and strength training "there seems to be a sort of bell curve of responsiveness; some quickly gain muscle or size, and others are fated never to progress, no matter how hard they try" (228).[19] This fact raises ethical questions that have not been fully studied since, as Kolata argues, "genetic testing and its psychological effects has focused on more profound questions" (229). As scandals involving steroids continue to develop, further studies of the ethics around performance-enhancing drugs will, no doubt, open other conversations about genetics and fitness. The toned ideal of the "perfect body," Kolata notes, "depends on whether one is genetically capable of building muscle and whether one is thin enough for the muscle to show" (234). We can see the ways in which our genes shape us and while we may not be able to change our genes, we can certainly navigate among the obstacles and find individual and structural ways to be healthy.

Balance and Flexibility

In life I find little balance
Giving too much of myself
To too many worthy causes
Sacrificing sleep to work
Relaxation to inspiration
Seeking a happy medium
Between have to and want to —

In life I have much flexibility
Bending over backward
For anyone I love
Or for expectations

Making adjustments
Accommodating last-minute
Changes and challenges
Stretching myself too thin —

In fitness classes
I have little flexibility
Stretching toward my comfort zone
And beyond is mostly impossible
The push and pull refuse to give instead

Finding balance
Stability with ease
Rooting myself
With purpose —
A foundation

— sometimes teetering
Always reaching...
then settling
for fitness and for life —
edges
of body and mind.

Balancing the Mind and Body: A Path Toward Healing

"The difficulties involved in women becoming fit are not only about self-image and self-worth, but considerations of time and money, alongside poor facilities and demanding family responsibilities. The balancing act of working women is finally being acknowledged as detrimental to health...."
— Tara Brabazon, "Fitness Is a Feminist Issue" (77)

"Yoga is learning to come back to yourself. It's finding your limits, expanding your boundaries, and being able to truly relax into who you are. It's about taking time to remember who you are but have forgotten while being caught up in the whirlwind of fast-paced life."
— Christina Brown, *The Yoga Bible* (8)

"'To lose balance sometimes for love is part of living a balanced life.'"
— Wayan, as quoted by Elizabeth Gilbert in *Eat, Pray, Love* (298)

"This conversation around the relationship between internal and external transformation will undoubtedly continue as more and more people feel the urge to bring a world out of balance back to equilibrium."
— Be Scofield, "Yoga for War: The Politics of the Divine" (149)

Yoga-related documentaries and memoirs capture the appeal of yoga as a means to find ourselves — to find balance if not deeper meaning. In

Enlighten Up! A Skeptic's Journey into the World of Yoga, filmmaker Kate Churchill "is determined to prove that yoga can transform anyone." Such a search for meaning is often done from a position of privilege, at least when taken up by North Americans and Europeans; we need to *process*. We need to believe in something. We need to believe we can be transformed. We need something to help us make sense of so many contradictions. This is the case for *Yoga Is: A Transformational Journey*. Suzanne Bryant finds her life changed when she learns of her mother's terminal cancer diagnosis and she finds that only her yoga practice (taken up previously to deal with New York anxiety) helps her to accept what is happening. She then explores what "yoga is" through a variety of themes — truth, happiness, the now, love — through interviews, and her own practice.

We also need the respite from our very busy, very distracted lives. We struggle with balance, letting go, living in the present. Perhaps the most well-known of such public introspection is Elizabeth Gilbert's *Eat, Pray, Love*, a *New York Times* bestseller that became a film starring Julia Roberts. Gilbert's search for balance takes her inside and outside herself. She finds "this happy, balanced *me*" (329) through a year-long process filled with mysticism, self-exploration, and an extended community of friends she makes along the way. She finds this balance, ultimately, through love.

* * *

Some of us are so unhappy (with ourselves, our lives, our jobs, etc.) that exercise simply brings us back into balance; it makes us almost able to function as if we were balanced happy people. And for some, happiness overflows in a saccharine bubbly river. Too much caffeine, like too much sugar or too much training supplement can leave us with an extra store of what might be mistaken for happiness. Gina Kolata explores the idea of the "runner's high," a euphoria that "can vary enormously from person to person" (191) and is rather vague in how it is achieved and experienced aside from involving "endorphins" (177). Ultimately, the happiness that exercise brings us (or can bring us) is a feeling of well-being, a balance of body and mind, "being able to truly relax into who you are." Exercise — getting the heart pumping on the treadmill or slicing through the water — might bring us endorphins, a moment like happiness. Fitness with mindfulness brings us a sustained balance of endorphins along with a wealth of benefits. The fact that Gina Kolata's *Ultimate Fitness* ends on the note of pleasure speaks to the possibilities of this less-recognized power of exercise. But pleasure is a beginning. In *Eat, Pray, Love*, Liz is looking for a different balance of pleasure and devotion (30).

Here, yoga is aligned with devotion, and yoga certainly plays a role in helping to restore some semblance of balance in her life.

The power of fitness to balance the body and mind has not gone unnoticed by mental health care providers — psychologists, psychiatrists, counselors, therapists, nurses, and doctors have used fitness, generally, and yoga specifically, to help clients better their health and quality of life. The nursing program at my university incorporates yoga into its curriculum. Counselors suggest approaches to health and fitness before, or in addition to medications. In *21st Century Yoga*, the authors "collectively illustrate how yoga can help heal some of the most devastating afflictions ravaging our society today including negative body image, disordered eating, and drug addiction" (xii). Lesley University in Massachusetts, as well as other universities and programs, offer expressive therapies and movement therapies as a part of their counseling programs. Books like *Yoga as Medicine: The Yogi Prescription for Health and Healing* provide an overview of various ailments and yogic practices that can counteract them. Author, Timothy McCall, M.D., writes in the introduction about how his first encounter with yoga was "in the same spirit" that he might try other activities, as simply "something interesting I'd heard about and decided to try." But he finds much more with yoga: "My body has changed in ways I wouldn't have believed possible, as has my mental state.... I didn't come in with any kind of faith that yoga would change my life, but it did" (xv). As fitness and yoga become better known approaches to healing, they will become less chastised as "alternative" forms of healing and medicine and more respected as preventetive.

Another book, *Emotional Yoga: How the Body Can Heal the Mind* provides a way of understanding the role of emotions in our mind/body fitness pursuits. Bennett writes, "yoga is a methodology for helping you access, transform, and heal your emotions, as well as your body and mind.... Ultimately, it will help you to heal yourself" (xv). Bennett makes a compelling case for the practice of "Emotional Yoga," beyond the expected arguments of dealing with stress or maintaining health or emotional balance. She writes, "Emotional Yoga involves your whole life" (xviii) and she argues that "you *can* change how you feel" and "there *is* something you can do about it" (author's emphasis). Thus, Emotional Yoga fosters empowerment, a more developed sense of self, and the permission to "become an active force in designing your health" (xix). Ultimately, Emotional Yoga is not simply about the individual, though this is certainly the starting point: Emotional Yoga "opens your possibilities of how to live and act in the world, and gives you the chance to experience what really matters — life itself" (xix).

My personal experience, and the anecdotal experience shared with me, speaks to the healing power of yoga and other forms of movement. Bennett offers some interesting perspective on movement and emotion, more general than yoga: "emotion means 'energy in motion,' and emotional energy is creative energy.... As we move, we feel, and as we feel, we experience inner and outer movement of our bodies and minds" (xv). I hear testimony nearly every day about physical healing: ankles, shoulders, and backs (almost as often as I hear testimony about injuries). These benefits are most noticeable in yoga or other mind/body fitness practices. While perhaps one of the most difficult benefits of yoga to measure through science, Broad finds that the ways in which yoga impacts mental health are certainly some of yoga's more legitimate claims. He witnesses yoga's transformative impacts on one of his interviewees, Amy Weintraub, whose yogafordepression.com provides a resource and a portal to her particular brand of LifeForce Yoga meant to "manage mood." LifeForce Yoga "is Yoga plain and simple. It doesn't really need a name, but in this day and age, when there are so many ways of practicing that are called Yoga, it's important to identify a practice that is intentionally designed to work with and manage the mood" (Amy Weintraub). Even within the confines of branded American fitness, "yoga plain and simple" is powerful.

Robert Downey Jr., featured in yoga poses in a 2012 *Men's Fitness Magazine* cover story, also cites yoga as being a positive and transformative effect in his life, a transformation that has resurrected his career and stayed his problems with addiction. A 2008 *TIME Magazine* article describes him as "Back from the Brink" and notes how he is "mellow and reflective after a morning of power-flow yoga with his teacher Vinnie Marino." Yoga is also credited in the recovery of Jason Russell, who experienced one of the most infamous public breakdowns when his KONY 2012 video went viral. Russell withdrew from the public eye for a period as he tried to recover. Later, he said: "I mean, it's hard for my wife to even talk about it still, because it was so scary and traumatizing." He continues, "It's just been really spending time with my family, a lot of slowing down, yoga, therapy. It's really been healing for the mind, body, and soul." Lady Gaga agrees too. According to an April 2013 article on celebuzz.com, "Gaga has admitted that with [Bikram studio owner Tricia] Donegan's help, she has healed her body, ever since her pre-fame college years." The article also notes that yoga has been cited for helping the pop star "monster" with physical and mental healing and "for her, there's no place like yoga to help her mind and body," which has helped to inspire her new movement, "A Body Revolution 2013." In these examples, mind/body transformations are visible and public.

Even without the mandates of mental health experts or celebrities, yoga is a way of working through emotions, obstacles, and fears — through life. This is exactly what Clair Dederer does in her yoga memoir, *Poser: My Life in Twenty-Three Yoga Poses.* She writes, "yoga for me was an attempt to fix something that was wrong with me. This anxiety that I didn't understand, that seemed to come from nowhere" (106). Whether we appreciate the ways in which Dederer makes sense of her life, or we find ways of thinking about our own lives (or both), yoga provides a kind of introspective map, if we want to follow it. As Dederer notes in the first few lines of her prologue: "taking up yoga in the middle of your life is like having someone hand you a dossier about yourself. A dossier full of information you're not really sure you want" (3). Throughout the book she reads her body to discover her emotions. The tight feeling in her chest while finding camel pose — fear — and her struggles to find her core while in warrior II lead to her finding not her "spiritual warrior," but her "real warrior," realizing that she was "spoiling for a fight" (172). She recognizes the power of mountain pose: "heavy, inert, solid, intractable. These are not things women are supposed to be" (253). Yoga is both literal — breathing, lifting, bending — and figurative; and she weaves between the postures of yoga class and the (rather mundane) obstacles of her life in "a North Seattle neighborhood filled with educated, white, liberal, well-intentioned people" (7). [20] Her journey through these twenty-three poses also takes her back through the struggles of growing up, piecing together a healing that bridges the past and present as well as the physical and mental.

While "fitness" usually considers cardio and strength as important components, and yoga links the mind, body, and emotions, the importance of sleep is less often seen as a factor in our overall fitness. Some experts argue that sleep is integral to optimal fitness. And better sleep is another benefit of regular fitness. More than sleep, we might neglect the importance of ease. New studies, captured by internet headlines, remind us to "Go Easy on Yourself, A New Wave of Research Urges." Beating ourselves up mentally and physically takes its toll. As Tara Parker-Pope writes, "the research suggests that giving ourselves a break and accepting our imperfections may be the first step toward better health ... [which] is not to be confused with self-indulgence or lower standards." This article is particularly focused on the importance of "self-compassion" as it relates to fitness, specifically to eating habits. As Parker-Pope notes, a 2007 study done by researchers at Wake Forest University "suggested that even a minor self-compassion intervention could influence eating habits." Giving ourselves permission to eat what we want to eat, rather than berating ourselves when we eat something that is "unhealthy," might be a better strategy to overall weight management. In this study, "the women who gave themselves permission to enjoy the sweets didn't overeat." Since "emotional eating" is a challenge for many of us, perhaps "self-compassion" can help to balance or redirect our emotions.

The importance of "self-compassion" and "self-care" (at its base: self-love) should not be overlooked, but pursuing a life free from stress might not be possible, let alone desirable. As much as stress can take a toll on our bodies, stress might also help us to achieve our goals and stay focused and motivated. In her article, "Can Stress Really Be Good for You?" MSNBC health editor, Jane Weaver, discusses some of the ways in which researchers are discovering the possible positive impacts of "moderate amounts" of stress, liked improved memory. She writes: "Good stress is the type of emotional challenge where a person feels in control and provides some sense of accomplishment. It can improve heart function and make the body resistant to infection, experts say. Far from being something we need to eliminate from our lives, good stress stimulates us." Her argument here is interesting; it seems we need moderate or "good stress" in order to succeed at our goals and protect our bodies from illness. Of course, like anything, too much stress is not good. Weaver notes, "the key is channeling stress energy into productive action instead of feeling overwhelmed, experts say." Clearly, balance is once again a factor in finding mind/body fitness. And as much as we use exercise to combat stress, one doctor that Weaver quotes points out that exercise itself "elevates stress hormones in the body and, through its cardiovascular benefits, actually makes the brain and body more resistant to psychological stress." So, if moderate stress, accessed through moderate exercise can make us more resistant to psychological stress, then we have found yet another therapeutic benefit to exercise.

Like any other forms of therapy, we have to want to be healed by movement in order for such remedies to be successful. McCall reminds us that "yoga is not a panacea, but it is powerful medicine indeed for body, mind, and spirit" (xix). The failure of yoga or movement to heal is about more than just the placebo effect at work or New Age healing promises exposed as frauds. Simply participating in a form of movement without engaging the mind, might not have the full range of potential effects. Likewise, there might just be mental illnesses that cannot be healed by the magic of movement, particularly without consent from the body and mind engaged in, or disengaged from, the practice. McCall continues, "Above all, yoga is a path. The longer you stay with it and the more heart you put into the journey, the farther it can take you" (xix). Even as I site my own observations, and those of others, there is no miracle that yoga specifically, or fitness generally, holds, no innate transformative power. We can't force a particular outcome or hope for a particular end result. As Claire Dederer writes toward the end of her yoga memoir, *Poser: My Life in Twenty-three Yoga Poses*, "I thought I would do yoga all my life, and I thought that I would continue to improve at it, that I would penetrate its deepest mysteries and finally be able to perform a transition from scorpion directly into chaturanga. But here's the truth: The longer I do yoga, the worse I get at it. I can't tell you what a relief it is" (329). In letting go, we are making room to move.

Fitness Saves Lives

"Yoga can kill and maim — or save your life and make you feel like a god. That's quite a range. In comparison, it makes most other sports and exercise seem like child's play."
— William J. Broad, *The Science of Yoga* (10)

"Feminism and yoga raised my consciousness and led me back to myself in love. The distorted image in the mirror had been shattered. I attribute these two complimentary systems for suturing the emotional and physical wounds and saving my life."
— Melanie Klein, "How Yoga Makes You Pretty: The Beauty Myth, Yoga and Me" (40)

I have heard many stories about the ways in which fitness saved someone's life. William Broad tells such success stories, as do the testimonials of participants of every fitness form from CrossFit to weightlifting to running to Zumba to Nia. A stark example is offered on the PostSecret website, "an ongoing community art project where people mail in their secrets anonymously on one side of a homemade postcard." On one such card, written in black marker over a montage of headless, muscled magazine man bodies an anonymous postcard reads: "the only thing stopping me from killing myself is my next workout." Whether it is through a recognition of one's personal power, a job in a tough economy, a philosophy that finally exhumed the demons of an eating disorder, dealing with devastating loss, or the physical and mental strength to overcome domination, fitness can saves lives in many different ways — in reality or metaphor. And fitness saved my life in a way that I rarely share with people, publicly or privately.

* * *

When I was a freshman in college I gained quite a bit of weight. I gained it slowly through an overindulgence in the readily available supply of junk food in the cafeteria and in the access of a credit card (later debt) and a friend's car. We would frequent El Torito for tortilla soup and quesadillas, the convenience store for pints of Ben & Jerry's (eaten in one sitting), and food was a central entertainment. I would drink several glasses of milk with dinner and treat myself to dessert at every meal. I had no regular activity to do and no one to do any activity with, and I spent most of my time reading and working on the school newspaper, pulling all-nighters fueled by candy and caffeine.

A few times I forced myself to go for a walk. My already-tight fitness clothes were tighter, and my regular clothes just didn't fit right. Because I had always considered myself to be fat, I did not realize that I was slowly becoming fat. I felt like my body was finally reflecting who I really was and did not realize that my body was quite different than it had been. When I changed schools my sophomore year and moved in with my boyfriend, I began to realize that I was unhappy with myself. I began to see that after years of *thinking* I was fat, now I really was fat. I opted for baggy clothes and withdrew from meeting new people. I was shy and insecure, and, at 19, I was younger than most of the people I met at work, at school, and in my neighborhood.

I don't remember what the specific catalyst finally was. I only remember that I finally decided that I no longer wanted to be fat. Childhood friends dropped by for a surprise visit, and I could find nothing to wear. And, generally, I felt that what I looked like on the outside was not matching how I felt on the inside. I finally decided that I was going to lose weight, and my mom supported me by offering to pay for a weight-loss system — supplements from Herbalife. Through some combination of supplement and determination, I drastically changed my diet. But I did not exercise. I lost a substantial amount of weight in ways that I would not recommend to anyone; but it worked. And losing this weight is what gave me the confidence to begin to take some credit aerobics classes through my university. And this is when I found out about a semester-long fitness instructor training course. I took this course the last semester of my senior year of college, in part because I thought maybe I could teach fitness part-time in between my undergraduate education and graduate school. I had it all planned out; my own version of a white picket fence.

I was driven through, and throughout, college. I had it all together academically (I thought). I did not have it all together personally, emotionally, spiritually. I had no idea to pay attention to such distractions. I did not know myself (as much as I thought that I did) and barely, but continually, pushed at the edges of what I thought I *should* do. One thing that had been ingrained in me from a very early age was that I *should* get married. This seemed to be the end-all point to life, and I thought that marriage was the relationship solve-all, that if you got married your problems went away. You were in it for the long haul, committed, invested. I take commitment seriously, and so I also took this expectation of marriage seriously even though it wasn't like this demand came directly from my parents or my friends. Mostly it came from the cultural messages that I took to heart uncritically or, rather, as a way of being and feeling normal, of being and doing what was expected of me, of proving I was loved. Getting married was a logical next step to life and love; it was autonomy from my parents as much as it was a new familial responsibility.

After getting married, we moved to Oregon and I started graduate school. My husband was unemployed and I decided to focus on school and not teach fitness classes. Teaching fitness was a distraction from my real, serious work (I thought), the work that was crucial to my future. I took some classes but found it difficult to keep up with more than one or two fitness classes a week. There was work to be done and my personal life at home was making less and less sense.

My husband was depressed (I realized later) but also deeply unaware of this depression, and I certainly did not know enough to recognize depression as a problem. I had never experienced it, and I had never been told about its existence as a problem in many people's lives. The quirks in his personality, the signs of abuse I could not see clearly before, began to manifest themselves in verbal, and eventually, physical abuse and violence. I was in a bad place that got worse. And I had no self-esteem. I had no support network. I had no insight. The small signs manifested themselves into one horrible night, a nightmare. I escaped my house — I had enough sense to pack up some important belongings (mostly my school work for the semester since it was the beginning of finals week). But he found me across town at a friend's house, and I had to call the police. The nightmare continued as I was questioned and manipulated by the police, as my bruises were photographed with a Polaroid camera. I was finally directed to the local shelter, a resource that I did not know existed. I was a shell. A *hard* shell.

I wanted to find my own way — our own way — but the courts were able to dictate my/our healing process. Some of the resources provided/mandated were helpful, but a better support system that would let me have power and find empowerment (rather than treating me like a victim and forcing me to pay fines for the crimes committed against me) would have been more helpful. Nothing made sense any more, least of all myself. I had been hollowing myself out for months. I had been floating along. I was determined that I would not be the victim that my husband, and then the police and the system, had created. I would be a survivor. I would find myself again. I only spent one night at the shelter but its existence is a continuing source of comfort and motivation. I was not like the other women who were there; but I was *one of them.* I am one of them. And I will always be one of a billion women impacted by violence.

As I began to rebuild my life, the most important work I had to do was to rebuild myself. Fitness was a major tool in this process. I decided that I would start teaching fitness classes again and that I needed to work out on a regular basis in order to deal with stress and in order to have my own space and place. I began teaching fitness classes and quickly began teaching other people how to teach fitness classes. My self-esteem grew and as my body got stronger, I became stronger. I marked my body, first with a belly button piercing and next with a tattoo, symbols of my strength and of the power contained within my body. My husband remembered my strength — not as a threat, but as an integral part of me that he loves. He had to heal too. And we had to heal together. We had to try to keep growing together as well. It has not been easy; old demons continue to scratch at the edges, threatening the mind, if not the body.

Love — in all its forms — is not easy. Sometimes fitness is the only thing that holds me together. It is consistent and evolving, distraction and decompression. My life has been built upon a foundation of fitness that is about more than just the body. And it is about more than just the mind. The fact that fitness is about a better body is an important point. This "better" body is not better because it fits with patriarchal, white supremacist standards as American popular culture, for instance, tells us. This body is better because it helps me to do what I want to do. It reminds me to remain steady, to find balance. It reminds me to never sacrifice myself to an unattainable ideal. It reminds me that I am powerful and strong in spirit and mind. It reminds me that transformation is possible.

FIVE

Transformations

From "Fitness" to Mind/Body Fitness

"*Movement Must Be Conscious, Not Habitual.* Whole-being fitness begins with heightened awareness — of both body and mind."
> — Debbie Rosas and Carlos Rosas,
> *The Nia Technique* (17; original emphasis)

"These images [of strong women] place too much hope in the transformational powers of individuals and they rely too heavily on the physical body as a resource of change. In doing so, they make three of the most general mistakes of capitalism: they hide labor, ignore history, and erase community."
> — Jacqueline Brady, "Beyond the Lone Images
> of the Superhuman Strongwoman..." (80)

While we have been considering fitness and feminist fitness, generally and specifically, we have also been exploring mind/body fitness — a connection between our physical and intellectual, emotional and critical selves, a connection between thinking and feeling — a connection that American culture often severs before it can even be explored. The concept of connections between mind and body are certainly not new, ancient philosophies (East and West) explore this dichotomy (or union). The mind/body connections are clear in many of the fitness forms and theoretical lenses I consider throughout this book.

These mind/body connections are not where the fitness industry has focused during its expansion and specialization phase of the 80s and 90s. Only with the recent boom of yoga and other mind/body forms of exercise has the fitness industry began to recognize that there may be value (and, thus, profit) in more conscious forms of exercise. But we might question whether the "fitness industry" is the best manager of mind/body fitness. The fact that William J. Broad focuses so much attention on the "waves of injuries" (10) that have supposedly resulted from yoga means that yoga's power to draw awareness inward, to connect the mind and the body, is not always heeded in yoga practice. If yoga is practiced without setting aside one's ego, by undertaking extreme practices, is it really yoga? If it's practiced in isolation, without connections off the mat, is it yoga? Maybe, but is it really mind/body feminist fitness?

The injuries that have resulted from yoga's boom are similar to the injuries that resulted from the boom of aerobics in the 80s. According to Debbie Rosas and Carlos Rosas, early injuries in aerobics (circa 1983) indicated "the human leg just isn't built for the pounding of conventional aerobics, including long-distance jogging" (14). While low-impact forms of aerobics have been developed, the same kinds of myths that promote the appearance of the body over the function of the body, have perpetuated the myth that low-impact means low intensity and a sub-par workout. Low impact can be an intense cardio workout. Modifications of movements are not necessarily transformative unless they also modify our minds — the way we think about the movements that we are doing.

In the early 1980s, as Debbie and Carlos recognized the importance of this shift, they also recognized that the conventional exercises they had been doing and teaching were inadequate for overall, functional fitness. As they encountered martial arts they found that there was a disconnect between how they were told to move and how they were able to move. They argue, "all our repetitive exercises had programmed us neurologically for rigid, mechanical movements, something very common among exercisers" (14–15). This mind/body connection, this programming is not a common way to think about fitness. We are not likely to equate, for instance, a rigidity in our fitness routine to rigidity in our ability to adapt to changes in our lives. Our understandings of fitness movements are literal. Debbie and Carlos suggest that as we embark into mind/body exercise programs like Nia we "should also stop performing conventional repetitive exercises, because they limit movement choices, reinforce robotic living, and often lock in mental and spiritual blocks" (17). A spectrum of movement choices are best for overall fitness. Perhaps this variety might supplement "robotic living" if not transform "mental and spiritual blocks."

This way of thinking about fitness does not have to be particular to a program. Shifting our attention to mind/body fitness as the basis of fitness means that any exercise we approach can be mind/body fitness; however, we need a critical framework for fitness that helps us make sense of our movement and, by extension, our physical, mental, emotional lives. If it is true, as Debbie and Carlos argue, that "psychologically, ... the militaristic, punishing element often found in traditional fitness ... creates resistance and insecurity, rather than enthusiasm and self-respect" (18), then it makes sense that those of us most wedded to traditional fitness practices would be most skeptical and may even fear the benefits promised by mind/body fitness. If the results of our fitness programs, routines, and practices are "enthusiasm and self-respect," then mind/body fitness promises plenty of other rewards as well.

Pirkko Markula's chapter in *Women and Exercise*, "'Folding': A Feminist Intervention in Mindful Fitness," is an important consideration of this shift from fitness to mind/body fitness or, "mindful" fitness as she refers to it. A mindfulness approach includes "'being present' during the activity, process orientation, slowness and embracing the activity itself" (60). Markula notes the rise in mindful forms of fitness, namely yoga, Pilates, and Tai Chi, but also hybrid forms. She also notes that mindful concepts are being incorporated into other kinds of fitness classes like step or strength training (60). She explains that "mindful fitness aims to bring the 'mind' back into the gym to provide more meaningful and varied exercise practices" (62).

In the project she details here she offers several examples of her approach to making feminist interventions through a Pilates class she taught for one hour, once a week, for twelve months. In this class she: "made a concerted effort never to mention the looks of the body"; emphasized connections to everyday movement; used music in the background "not to create an army of uniform exercisers (as might be the case in aerobics classes)"; incorporated modifications into beginner classes aimed toward progressing; "shared knowledge with participants rather than simply ordering them to do one exercise after another"; "dressed in loose clothing instead of revealing, tight exercise wear"; "avoided demonstration" so that clients would concentrate on their own movement, not try to imitate the instructor; and used touch to "[awaken] some bodily feelings" (68–74). All of these are important practices that might be executed differently depending upon the instructor, the time, the place, and the participants. For instance, for Markula, fighting the assumption of the "perfect body" might have come from wearing loose clothes, but for me, this intervention comes from wearing clothes that are optimal for movement (tight) and that most often reveal just how not perfect my body is. Further, it can be just as powerful an intervention to use music that inspires and informs movement rather than just keeping it as "background."

The interventions that Markula describes and analyzes are version of what I do — and every other conscious, committed, sometimes feminist instructor does — in our classes. Thus, I wonder if some of the challenges that Markula encountered were, at least in part, shaped by her approach as much as by the assumptions that exercisers held. For instance, she chooses not to demonstrate exercises and admits that "my clients were often confused with only verbal instruction"; she justifies this confusion saying, "but at the very least they had to concentrate on their movement execution instead of mechanically following me" (72). This is, in my experience, irresponsible instruction; she makes assumptions about what her demonstration might mean. She decides upon her approach in isolation from what the participants might need or want. She lets theory dictate practice. If a participant is unsure about how to do something, it will be difficult for her to feel her body, to connect her mind and her body. Discomfort, confusion, fear of failure, anxiety, and injury can all result from this approach. Further, there is no reason why modeling movement would interfere in participants' connections of mind and body or their ability to feel. In fact, verbal cues, especially without visual or kinesthetic cues, can make it just as difficult to focus on our own bodies and movements. Critical instructors know that they have to use a variety of methods to reach all of the different people in their group fitness classes.

She also ran into problems when participants complained that they wanted to "'work harder'" because "they did not 'feel anything'" (70). It is a challenge to get participants to perceive mind/body exercise differently from other fitness forms. Rather than find a way to show participants what the "work" of class was, she "ended up providing more advanced modifications so that the clients could work harder although they did not possess the skills to do such modifications yet" (70). From an instructor's perspective, this is the short-term, easy way out. I've taken it myself at times. Participants who don't listen to the alternatives and variations, and when and how these should be done, is another challenge that I deal with in virtually every class I teach. They think that they need to, for instance, touch the floor in Triangle pose by bending forward or hold their arms over head in Warrior I despite a shoulder injury. I constantly emphasize choosing the "best options for you today" and repeat over and over again the importance of listening to your body. I do the "easy" options and sometimes stay there. Even so, there are always those participants who lean forward out of alignment to reach the floor or take the high impact options every time because they think that the low impact options are less intense. Markula found that "teaching the participants to 'feel' their bodies presented the most challenging task, particularly against the powerful notions of hard work and continuous progression" (71). This is *the* challenge of mind/body fitness instruction *and* practice.

Ultimately Markula argues that "We need to think about the meaning of the movement, not copy pre-established patterns. We need to teach participants to feel the movement, to find their own rhythm, to find their own bodies" (75). Fitness instructors of all kinds are experimenting with ways to do this. And there are plenty of instructors, participants, and programs that adhere to the patterns established by manufactured as well as organic programs. In both cases, these methods are largely divorced from academia and are isolated from other instructors' attempts. Markula notes that teaching Pilates is a "more active feminist intervention" (60) than her work in academia. Finding ways to merge spheres and shrink distance are key to critical mind/body transformations.

* * *

The last part of this book considers individual and structural transformations of all kinds, and I transform topics discussed previously. Here I consider what developing consciousness might mean in relation to fitness, how this kind of development is more than just a mind/body connection, and how fitness can provide a path to mind/body empowerment. I relate many of my transformative fitness experiences like discovering the power of dance as well as how these movements and practices have changed my fitness practice as well as my life. I explore how my teaching has been transformed by considering the differences between instruction and performance and the ways in which changing direction in the fitness studio changed my perspective as well.

In this section I also critically consider fitness spaces that need more critical attention in order to lead to individual and structural transformation. For instance, I consider the predominance of whiteness and economic privilege and other cultural barriers that keep people from practicing fitness and pursuing a kind of fitness that is different from, challenges, and even transforms mainstream fitness definitions and expectations. I attempt to move American fitness ideas and practices toward feminist mind/body fitness ideas and practices. Such a shift requires all kinds of transformations.

Sketches: Transforming Local and Docile Bodies and Minds

The sketches throughout this book speak to the power of transformative innovators as well as the lived experiences of fitness instructors and participants. In this last installment I focus on transformation on the local level — the space where most of us experience fitness — in order to highlight the ways in which individuals are able to make transformations of all kinds in their lives and the lives of others. But I also focus on the structural, a system of institutions that socializes us to be docile bodies — to contain our lived experiences in order to fit into the roles that society has arranged. Docile bodies need to have docile minds; oppositional minds make rebellious bodies. Here too, the efforts of transformative innovators — of individual workers and community initiatives — negotiate the edges of fitness toward transformation at the individual and structural levels. The transformations sketched out here speak to several possibilities for individuals and communities, systems and structures.

Local Incarnations: Valance and Kaya Fitness

Val Kitchen is not world-famous. She does not own a training system, a patent, a line of DVDs, or a multi-million dollar business. In fact, she regularly attends trainings, learns new skills, and purchases new equipment. She likes to keep moving, and she likes to find ways to keep her clients moving as well. Val Kitchen is a pillar of her community in Bangor, ME, a founding presence in aerobics, and a transformative innovator on a variety of levels.

Val is a bundle of energy and she almost literally never stops. She takes her work seriously and has a passion for exercise and for providing a service to people in order to enhance their lives and abilities. After more than 30 years teaching and developing programming at the YMCA/YWCA, Val opened her own studio in downtown Bangor. Everyone knows Val and Val knows everyone. The first time I tried to find her studio I asked someone where I could find Valance studio and she answered, pointing, "Oh, Val's place. It's right there." And when I have walked/talked with Val on sunny afternoons, she greets many people she knows. When she doesn't know you, she'll talk to you anyway. And she is genuine. Valance Pilates, Fitness, and Dance Studio expresses her passion and skills.

While Val went out on her own after years of service at the YWCA/ YMCA, many young women (and men) are opening their own gyms and fitness studios. As Amanda Vogel argues in an article in *IDEA Fitness Journal* about Generation X and the future of fitness, "the second wave of fitness pros continues to move the industry forward" (30). Creator of Kaya Fitness out of Pullman, Washington, Danielle Eastman, has held several different types of fitness positions; she earned her Master's in Exercise Physiology and she is a certified health and fitness specialist through ACSM. I first met her when she was my supervisor at the Washington State University's Student Recreation Center. She left shortly thereafter to pursue her own interests in fitness and she taught Nia and yoga through community recreation. After I had moved away, Danielle opened her own studio, Bliss, "a peaceful movement sanctuary" and then developed Kaya Fitness which she describes on her website as "balancing simple feel-good choreography with free-form bliss, Kaya classes deliver physical conditioning, creativity, community, self-discovery, and personal expression through all kinds of barefoot movement danced to all kinds of music." This description describes what I teach with my own flavor; without a trademark, there is no one name for what we do.

Kaya Fitness is certainly inspired by Danielle's many other fitness interests and trainings, particularly Nia. However, in creating her own brand, she is able to own what she does in the studio. She is able to create and guide without being subject to a particular set of rules, and without paying licensing or franchising fees. Opening her own studio was the first step. She could own and control the space, creating exactly the environment where she could practice and teach. Creating her own programming is an extension of this space and expresses love of freedom and movement, expression and community. Kaya fitness is a successful fitness brand (and I mean this in many incarnations of these terms) because of the qualities that Danielle brings to her work; she is genuine, thoughtful, caring, committed, brave, creative, and innovative, and she connects with people, individually and in groups.

Danielle's technological skills support her fitness endeavors. Active on Facebook and Twitter, and with her own website, Danielle's message gets out wider than her Pullman community. The visual appeal of her site, its moving quality, and inclusion of a balance of information and images, draws the viewer in. Her "tips" give the beginner an introduction and the active participant a reminder of "why we do what we do." Kaya embodies much of what I believe to be true about fitness and what I hope others will discover for themselves. Danielle is, after all, one of my teachers. She explains:

> Kaya is about celebrating your body through all kinds of blissful movement. It is a place for you to move, let go, be free ... where you can forget yourself & find yourself ... a practice through which one can learn about fitness, self-discovery, self-expression, vulnerability, community, empowerment, authenticity, and pure bliss ... all from the inside-out. Ultimately, Kaya is about setting yourself free. I would love to share this practice with you!

Pullman was my home for years and because of transformative innovators like Danielle, it calls me back to one of my fitness homes.

Ericka Huggins and YogaEd: Yoga for Incarceration and Education

A featured SpeakOut! presenter, Ericka Huggins, is a wealth of knowledge and experience on a variety of subjects. On her official website she describes herself: "As an activist, former political prisoner & leader in the Black Panther Party, educator & student I've devoted my life to the equality of all — beyond

the boundaries of age, culture, class, gender, sexual orientation or ability."
Huggins's experiences are different from the other innovators I feature in this
book; however, the path that brought her to fitness is an important example
of American fitness. She adds an important political aspect to our understanding of American fitness as well as an important connection to community
values. While Huggins's work encompasses far more than just fitness, her
fitness-related projects echo her work in social justice, education, and creative
writing (poetry).

As a part of the Siddha Yoga Prison Project, beginning in 1979, Huggins
taught Hatha Yoga and meditation in California state and county prisons and
jails. She has continued such volunteer work, bringing yoga to youth and
adults in a variety of settings including homes for foster and adopted children
and pregnant teens as well as community colleges and Northern California
public schools, as her website bio explains. Ericka Huggins's work bringing
yoga to incarcerated populations is performed by many other far less famous
people in projects like Siddha Yoga Prison Project, part of an Ashram in Oakland, California, which aims to bring yoga to incarcerated individuals, or
Y.O.G.A. for Youth (Your Own Greatness Affirmed), which "provide[s] urban
youth with tools of self discovery that foster hope, discipline and respect for
self, others and community."

Huggins' work in prisons and with marginalized youth work is impressive; she took her skills to another context through her work from 1994
through 1999 as a training consultant and in-school educator for the
Mind/Body Medical Institute, an affiliate of Harvard Medical School. Her
website bio explains this work: "The program empowered teachers and students to practice relaxation, yoga stretching and mindfulness as a tool to
maintain internal locus of control and minimize daily challenges." Research
related to this work showed the positive impact that only a handful of visits
had on the youth in these programs, improving "standardized test scores,
school attendance and classroom management."

Yoga's benefits in educational settings are being explored and applied
through programs like Yoga Ed. or YoKids.org in Maine. Both of these programs aim to bring yoga into the schools and train teachers to incorporate
yoga into their classrooms. YoKids works at the local level, reaching out to
teachers in Maine and helping to implement yoga into around 30 schools,
day care centers, or programs in Maine. Yoga Ed. offers curriculum and training to yogis (people who have completed a yoga training program) and
provides "Yoga Tools for Teachers," a training that helps teachers use yoga
to teach students to "utilize simple yoga-based exercises to enhance health,
well-being, learning and responsible behavior." Yoga in schools has been

shown to curb the behaviors of bullying and is listed on Canada's Ministry of Education's Registry of Bullying Prevention Programs. Yoga Ed. has over 700 Yoga Ed. instructors and over 20 Yoga Ed. trainers, with its K–8 programs taught in more than 150 schools in 27 states. Yoga Ed. also has international programs as their influence reaches far and wide. Many of their trainers are amazing transformational innovators in their own right, founding programs for sexual assault awareness, yoga education, and national social action initiatives.

Clearly, Huggins's work as a transformative innovator has helped to lead the way in bringing yoga to incarcerated individuals and educational settings. As a professor of sociology and women's studies, she "brings her legacy of spiritual activism and social justice to her teaching." She also speaks widely on a number of topics, continuing to educate in and out of academia. These academic fields highlight the ironies of yoga in educational and carceral settings. One of the reasons that yoga has been accepted into prisons and schools is the assumption that yoga, as mind/body exercise is thought to, as Pirkko Markula explains, "create docile, productive, stress-free citizens" (64). Both prisons and schools are spaces where there is a desire for more docile subjects; both depend upon the obedience of their populations for a variety of reasons. Kids deal with more and more stress and have more distractions. They suffer from malnutrition and over-medication, food scarcity and obesity. We need them to sit still and learn and buy into their education. Prisoners are incarcerated for crimes that include those related to addiction, unemployment, hunger, and lack of educational opportunities. We need them to be docile so they are easier to control, and we need them to be productive because their slave labor provides us with many goods and services from Victoria's Secret underwear to the latest technological gadgets.[1] Markula asks, "is it possible to provide exercise practices that do not build docile bodies?" (64). In both settings, docility might be preferable, but another benefit of mind/body feminist fitness might be a greater capacity to think critically, to shift perspectives. Fitness might just be a means for challenging and transforming these institutional structures — education and incarceration.

The impact of yoga in schools has great transformative potential. As our concerns about safety and security in schools grow, we can see that these concerns echo our ideas of safety and security (and punishment and crime) in prisons. We react with more militarization, fences, rules, and less unstructured time. The relaxation techniques, sense of self, and other mind/body connections of feminist fitness might just be one part of an equation to increase safety *and* student success. But these are not the foci of our national agendas; they are the work of progressive, radical, often marginalized people.

Racing Cross-Cultural Connections

"Exercise is a luxury of time that few can afford. Because it is a scarce
resource, good health is a commodity, a lifestyle to be bought and
sold. The right to leisure is a new political battleground."
— Tara Brabazon, "Fitness Is a Feminist Issue" (72)

"Think about all of the white, middle- and upper-class people who
have been practicing yoga, meditating, doing visualizations, and
chanting in the West for decades now. Has it made them more aware
of injustice? More concerned about white privilege or informed about
racism? Better educated about poverty?"
— Be Scofield, "Yoga for War" (143)

Throughout this book I have explored a number of intersections that
speak to the whiteness of fitness — a dominance of white bodies as well as
white ideas, ideals, and politics. The seemingly *personal* goals of fitness can
seem like a luxury and/or a waste of time when there are bills to be paid, long
hours to be worked, children to shuttle from here to there, family demands,
dinner to be made. But food, water, clothing, shelter, education, healthcare,
and fitness are basic human necessities. And white people, in the U.S. and
around the world, continue to dominate the ownership and arrangement of
such resources. Conceptualizing fitness as a luxury relegates fitness to whiteness, to a kind of pure imaginary. It separates one's physical being from one's
emotional being; it assumes that fitness is a privilege rather than a right. When
we consider the global fitness trends, social class might be a more accurate
division of fitness — those who can afford to create and market and buy fitness
programs are overwhelmingly white. Whiteness is inescapable since historically
class and race are tied together. As Louise Mansfield and others note, the very
idea of the "better body" has its roots in white, middle-class, heterosexual
expectations of femininity and masculinity (88). As we better understand the
many dimensions and possibilities for fitness, we can begin to remake the
images, ideas, and ideals to better fit the many shades and variations of our
peoples.

Most of the skin I see on a daily basis (in my little geographic enclave)
is white and within this narrow array of racial tones there is a great diversity
in age, body type, income, sexuality, ethnicity, experience, confidence, ability,
personality, and interest. Regardless, most populations where I have taught
are predominantly (but not entirely) racially white; thus, my fitness population
is already demographically skewed. Fitness, on the level of instructors and
participants, is diverse in terms of race, gender, and sexuality according to
local and regional demographics, within the U.S. and around the world. Thus,

the "whiteness" of fitness is a cultural representation, an ideological description, and an individual participant identity. But fitness (and American pop culture more generally) does not need more tokenism or multicultural celebration; it needs a radical reconsideration.

Throughout this book I have offered a number of radical reconsiderations; here I turn to a radical reconsideration of the whiteness of fitness, of token representation or multi-cultural inclusion as a means to reinforce dominant ideologies. Fitness remains "white" in mainstream spaces even when Michelle Obama is an advocate or when it takes a tone of Hip Hop, for instance, as *LL Cool J's Platinum Workout* suggests or Shaun T's Hip Hop Abs displays. White enlightenment does not automatically equal concerns about justice, white privilege, racism, or poverty, as Scofield notes. We might begin to challenge narrow conceptualizations of "American fitness" by exploring marginalized voices and spaces. Simply adding color to a white pursuit or examining cultural representations and appropriations does not mean a radical reconsideration. We must dig deeper, look further, and adopt a critical lens.

* * *

Sharon Wray explains that "the current western-centric spotlight on individual and psychological influences on healthy behavior dangerously neglects how ethnicity and culture shape people's beliefs, views and behaviors" (176). This neglect is related to food and health, as well as to the overall approach to fitness and health promotions, undertaken by government and private entities. As Wray points out, "it is often assumed that people will change their 'health behaviors' if the health promotion interventions they are targeted with are cultural sensitive" (171). Of course, cultural sensitivity usually means that we (the powerful dominant culture) recognize that there are differences, and we celebrate your differences when they are convenient to us, but we are reaching out to you because we want you to know that there are better ways and we assume that if you know these better ways then you will want to adopt these ways.

In conversation with Amalia Mesa-Bains, bell hooks critiques these kinds of "conservative uses of multiculturalism" and argues that "progressives of all colors need to speak back" to these uses, "to simply recognize that a radical multiculturalism has never taken root in our cultural economy" (95). Thus, cultural sensitivity can be yet another means to dominate and oppress but "we are still in the process of creating theories of this radical multiculturalism" (95). Instead, a better approach might be, as Wray suggests, "to question how 'healthy' western ideas about healthy lifestyle are" (177) and, as bell hooks argues, "hopefully, as the theory is created, the praxis will emerge — a union of critical thinking and critical action" (95). Both the physical and mental health implications of dominant, mainstream fitness might be unhealthy if we change our lens. Radical reconsiderations of fitness, as well as radical reconsiderations of the power to define fitness for self or community, may happen in academia, but in the realm of Othered popular culture, the potential for radical reconsideration is ripe.

* * *

One of the best examples of a revolutionary approach to fitness through popular culture provides an interesting foil to the example of *LL Cool J's Platinum Workout*. Upon first glance or an initial listening to his album, *The Workout*, the work of rapper Khnum "Stic" Ibomu, may not seem to be that much different from what we find in *LL Cool J's Platinum Workout*. Both speak of a "paradigm shift" and speak to the importance of discipline and proper nutrition, though what constitutes such a shift and what's "proper" is vastly different (lean meats vs. a vegan diet, for instance). Both take a hard core, masculine workout approach that relies upon weight lifting and calisthenics even as they emphasize the importance of a stretching regimen. Both men are also black American rap artists; LL Cool J is credited with bringing "rap and hip-hop culture from the underground to the mainstream" (book jacket bio), and he has been firmly situated as a mainstream artist and celebrity ever since. Stic is best known for his work as a part of the "revolutionary hip hop duo dead prez" (web bio) which has remained "underground" even as elements of Stic's work filter into mainstream spaces like TV shows and collaboration with platinum-selling artists.

As a member of Dead Prez, Stic has challenged racism, white supremacy, imperialism, police brutality and corruption, and other ills of our white supremacist capitalist imperialist patriarchy (hooks) through his work for at least 20 years. [2] His music, both in the past and on *The Workout* speaks to a "warrior mentality" and the art of self-defense (both in a martial arts and Black Power context). RBG Fit Club, an online community founded by Stic, is creating a revolutionary approach to fitness, an online community, and a platform for a revolutionary fitness ideology and practice.[3] RBG Fit Club promotes the pillars of "knowledge, nutrition, exercise, rest, and consistency." This is "not a dogmatic program but a dynamic mindset," the RBG Fit Club website explains. The RBG fitness movement is an "engaging, motivational and culturally relevant movement" that is "authentically centered in hip hop culture," and speaks to the "urgency in our communities." Stic invites "people from all walks of life" to "enthusiastically take ownership of their health" so that they are "able to enjoy the benefits of healthy, energetic, prosperous and compassionate lives." RBG Fit Club then becomes a "collective example" that can "shift popular emphasis" and become a "powerful tool." Stic has also begun the Million Miles Movement, a "movement of the people" and a "community health initiative." The site argues: "This is a movement of the people; literally!" A collective raising of awareness, not only of the power of healthy diet and exercise but also of the potential of mass movement, "the strengthening of our collective will," is part of the purpose. And the effort of this RBG Fit Club initiative, and others, is to work "towards expanding the culture of healthier living." This culture is in direct conflict with mainstream America's ideas and ideals of "fitness."

Perhaps the most powerful means of disseminating his revolutionary approach to fitness, and the best way to understand the ways in which Stic's album differs from other celebrity approaches to fitness, is through the layered and powerful ideas that comprise *The Workout*. The album in its entirety speaks to a conscious, cross-training, whole body, and mind/body approach to fitness and casts a wide definition, even as it often relies upon common understandings of fitness in certain places like "no pain no gain" and a masculine universal approach. For instance, much of the album takes up the story of masculine icons like the warrior, the soldier, or the champion. (And two male icons — Bruce Lee and Joe Louis — have a song devoted to them.[4]) But he also complicates these icons. The champion, for instance, is not gendered and the soldier is "sober." This soldier stands as an example for the many people (male and female) who suffer from addiction; the "Sober Soldier" fights for families and communities impacted by the disease of addiction. The warrior too, is more complicated, drawing strength from the struggle.

Stic complicates ideas of masculinity in the ways I have described above but he also provides space on his album for an explicitly female (and perhaps feminist) perspective on fitness in the track "Baby Fat." While "Baby Fat" might be seen as a nod to the inclusion of the female perspective, the ideas expressed in this song and the way in which it is included is revolutionary, particularly when considered in comparison with the ways in which *LL Cool J's Platinum Workout* speaks to women. This song features the voices and lyrics of Maimouna Youssef, Afya Ibomu, and Ife Jie and offers a more complex look at the idea of "baby fat" as well as the ways in which women negotiate this concept through body and mind. The hook speaks to a more feminine approach to fitness. Strength, endurance, movement, and the ability to "work out" all kinds of things is encapsulated here. "Baby Fat" is not simply about getting rid of unattractive flesh, it's about a continuation of a level of fitness that was there before the baby came. Many of the women's lyrics might seem to speak to some of the mainstream expectations for women's fitness, but we cannot escape these expectations anywhere. Instead, this song provides a negotiation within this framework of the "beautiful body." The body is beautiful for what it can do — from workouts to having babies. Stic's part in the song is not dismissive of the work that goes into this process; instead, his words are a bolster, a reminder of the woman's own power. "Baby fat" is totally normal and temporary; the result of important women's work while also inconsequential to the woman and her work.

The Workout is not simply about gaining size (or losing baby fat) or becoming a warrior; it explores a variety of issues related to fitness including accessibility of fitness spaces, the need for discipline and purpose and balance, and a multi-pronged approach to one's workout. Part of dealing with the struggle and building fitness is practicing healthy eating. While considering what the body can achieve, he also examines what we put into our bodies (and minds), for instance, in the song "Healthy Livin'" where he promotes raw and vegan diet choices (as well as preventative health care). The healthy aspects of a vegan diet are still widely debated in and out of fitness circles, even when famous athletes prove its worth.[5] With all of the food myths that circulate, and all of the unhealthy choices that surround (and often define) us, both a fuller understanding and a means of educating our children are important toward a revolutionary shift in ideas about health, wellness, and fitness let alone justice and love. It is certainly an album that can complement a workout — an expansion of the mental and physical understandings of fitness. This is a power that holds potential for mind/body transformations.

Consumption and Control: Transforming Disordered Minds/Bodies

"I have that former-fat-kid thing of always waiting for the fat to come back and claim me. And this, of course, was one of the reasons I went to yoga. To barricade myself against the return of the fat. No one likes to talk about this aspect of yoga: It makes you thin. We were all supposed to be focused on breathing and being in the moment."
— Claire Dederer, *Poser: My Life in Twenty-three Yoga Poses* (199)

"What will you gain when you lose?"
— Special K commercials and ad campaign launched January 2011

"This is not just my legacy.... This legacy of low self-esteem and self-objectification — punctuated by disordered eating, continuous exercise, and abusive fat talk — keeps most girls and women stuck in an

unhealthy cycle that holds us back and prevents us from being truly empowered."
— Melanie Klein, "How Yoga Makes You Pretty:
The Beauty Myth, Yoga and Me" (29)

Dederer's struggles with feeling "fat" might be a surprise in a yoga memoir. As Dederer points out, weight loss is a controversial subject in yoga because of the more spiritual and mindful associations. But in Broad's estimate, yoga slows down metabolism and can cause weight gain, which undercuts those like Dederer who comes to yoga with that fat girl crying from inside, crumbling rather than employing Tiffany Kell's "Bendypants" tactics. After detailing several examples of "everything bad about my body that has ever been said to me," Dederer writes, "there are more. Obviously ... I am guessing that everyone has a list like this in their head — or every woman does. These feelings bring out a funny feeling (ha ha!) in me: guilt. Being fat, even a little bit fat, makes me feel guilty. My parents and brother are all very thin and so this is how I thought I ought to be" (198). Dederer identifies that these problems are cultural — connected to family and gendered expectations. Clearly these complicated issues mean that within mind/body fitness there is some movement to challenge "disordered" minds and bodies. In several sections of this book I have attempted to illuminate and unravel the tangled subject of "disordered eating." I have argued that disordered eating is part and parcel with our cultural values and promoted lifestyle. The links between fitness and perceived fitness based upon appearance are difficult to tease out. The links between food and fitness are entrenched and conflicted.

The structured inequalities of racism, sexism, and poverty are, of course, also layered with dominant ideas about fitness — what foods to eat or not eat, what exercises to do or not do, what bodies represent fitness and which do not. While not all fitness programs or fitness instructors will address food, Wray notes that "food is a symbol of identity so that eating particular foods signifies cultural tradition, values and collective identity boundaries" (174). Thus, the diet aspect of fitness can be a major stumbling block in terms of promoting fitness amongst those marginalized along the lines of race or class. The assumptions about what foods are healthy and which are not is often in direct conflict not only with cultural traditions or slim pocket books, but also with the very idea of what "fit" or "healthy" might mean. As Brabazon notes, "With the palate classed, so is the notion of fitness and leisure" (70).

Because food is an important aspect of health and fitness, and because women continue to hold primary responsibility for their family's food, it is important to consider the role that food might play in relation to culture. As Wray explains:

Historically and across culture, women have exhibited self-control about the types of foods they eat for reasons such as appearance, income, health, and spiritual and religious beliefs ... to an extent, control over the type of food that is eaten becomes a moral imperative that can only be maintained through acts of self-discipline. This moral control over the body may be experienced as empowering because it may equate with increased status within a particular community [175].

As Wray illustrates here, food has always been linked to "moral control" and "self-control" and women bear the brunt of these social and cultural imperatives. Thus, for the women in Wray's study, food was not simply about health and fitness, it was also about family and culture as well as individual choice and identity. Wray found that British and English participants in her study were more likely to conform to advice given by the instructor regarding food choices while Pakistani, British Muslim, and African Caribbean women "did not express a desire to adopt a western-centric healthy lifestyle" and "this resistance enabled the women to maintain religious and cultural collective identity boundaries" (176). The British and English women were conforming to cultural expectations about food (and self-control) as much as the women of color were conforming to their own cultural expectations. But the former would be considered "healthy," while the latter would not. Wray also found that this process of refusal was empowering to the women of color. Thus, we might consider how a different approach to diet, health, and fitness outreach might more effectively reach across cultural (racial and ethnic) boundaries.

Some mainstream corporations and campaigns embrace the idea of empowerment to varying degrees of success. For instance, Kellogg's Special K has long used the benefit of weight loss as a marketing tool. In 2011, an interactive Times Square event invited consumers to step on a large scale but rather than displaying a number, the scale displays an "inspirational word or phrase that captures the emotional benefit of achieving their goal," according to a news release. Launched with the new year, the associate director of the Special K brand, Jesper Lund Jacobsen, explains, "'we're looking to help reshape the mindset of how women approach weight loss in the New Year.'" Women participating in the Times Square event or the campaign more generally, had an opportunity to appear in commercials or to share their "gain" on product packaging or Facebook. Jacobsen explains that this "partnering" with women "'encourages women to focus on the positive *emotional* benefits that result from their efforts. We believe this additional support will ultimately help keep them motivated.'" Of course, this partnering is also a powerful way to promote the Special K Brand, a brand that is already connected to the idea of dieting.

In the U.S. we may rant against overconsumption and unrealistic images as much as we like, and sometimes we inspire transformation. Magazines like *BUST* give us historical perspective when they feature "vintage weight gain ads" with the headline "Skinny Girls Don't Have Oomph!" Websites like love-mybody.com can give us real-life comparisons and images of women. We may even succeed in small changes through campaigns and activism like Julia Blum and Izzy Labbe, Maine teens who challenged *Seventeen Magazine* to stop photo shopping their models (Laura Murphy). A website created by Emily Lauren Dick ("Average Girl"), loveaverage.com, provides an opportunity "for the Average Girl to begin talking about what really matters.... Where girls can challenge body and beauty image ideals and inspire each other to love the bodies they have!" Dick was a Women's Studies and Sociology major and is working on a book, *Average Girl: A Guide to Loving Your Body*. Her website provides images and commentary that illustrate the ways in which the media distort body image, but does so while providing positive ways of seeing ourselves and other women. A mix of celebrity quotes and feminist analysis, this site is an inspiration toward transforming dis-ordered minds/bodies.

Toward a more realistic body image, women in the industry are leading the way toward industry transformation like former model Katie Halchishick who initiated the "Healthy Is the New Skinny" campaign/movement/business and co-founded the non-profit Perfectly Unperfected Program (PUP) that brings this message to secondary schools and colleges. According to their website's "About Us" section, "Healthy Is the New Skinny **is a multi-platform movement** to bring a message of health, joy, and responsibility to the beauty and the fashion industries. Through bold and creative initiatives, HNS works with media, corporate, and modeling partners to create lasting change" (original emphasis). Such movements are a step in the right direction, but still emphasize outward appearance, even as a means to less superficial concerns. As the "Healthy Models" section of the PUP website states: "A critical part of the solution is offering counter images: models who exemplify beauty and vibrant good health across the size spectrum. This isn't just about 'Plus-Size' models: this is about promoting a new, attainable ideal for women regardless of natural body type. "Counter-images that are truly "every size" and "about celebrating looking good, feeling good, and doing well for life. At every size" are potentially revolutionary. How we interpret these more realistic images may still be skewed, but at least we are challenging the manufactured images that confront us on a daily basis, in a variety of places, on a variety of levels.

* * *

We can be hard on ourselves and alternately be empowered and free of judgment. We can change the way we see ourselves and others — our body image — this thing that only reflects a fragment of our bodies and even less of our minds. But this is a bigger social and cultural disease. As Tara Brabazon argues, "this disordered nature of eating — the compulsions, purging and binging — is embedded in the disordered nature of the political economy and hyperconsumerism" (69). Our issues with food are bigger than food. We can begin, on the individual level, by practicing mindful eating.[6] Developing a better, more conscious, and less judgmental relationship with food is an important aspect of mindful eating, also known as Intuitive Eating, as developed and described by Evelyn Tribole and Elyse Resch in their book *Intuitive Eating: A Revolutionary Program That Works.* A wealth of information is included on their website intuitiveeating.org — most immediately useful: 10 Principles of Intuitive Eating — and a 2012 edition of the book includes updates that consider kids and teens as well as the science behind Intuitive Eating. At its heart, listening to your body (and not to damaging cultural messages) is the key to this philosophy and practice.

Intuitive Eating has much in common with mindful fitness practices, and the two can be linked together in ways that challenge traditional weight loss approaches and strategies. Taking time to enjoy the experience of eating — the taste and feel of food, eating for nourishment and hunger, for health and wellness — can make a change in the ways in which we approach food and our overall fitness. These are not new ideas. Health and fitness crusaders have been urging us to practice these ways for over a century (Wharton). When we decide to listen and practice both eating and exercising more mindfully, we are tapping into the potential for transformation on a larger scale than our individual health and fitness. We are challenging long-standing American ideologies. Thus, we might also think about this concept of mindful eating in relation to what we consume more generally. Mindful eating is one approach to eating disorders like binge eating and overeating as well as anorexia and bulimia. Mindless consumption or steadfast control are at the heart of these disorders, just as this quality is at the heart of American consumerism.

* * *

It is impossible to pursue fitness without also consuming products, advice, and fuel, but this does not mean that consumption needs to be excessive or exploitative. Purchasing the latest diet fad, the most expensive clothing, the trendiest accessories, the most talked-about program, the highest quality foods and supplements, are certainly examples of American patterns of obsessive consumption and the American problem of consumerism. We like "cheap, accessible and fast" (Brabazon). This kind of consumption is a larger problem in the U.S. generally; and within the fitness industry specifically, many companies try to make products toward more mindful fitness and more mindful consumption practices. Ultimately, however, consumption is the responsibility of the consumers and collective initiatives are central. Doing more with less need not be a mantra of only the oppressed or the arrogant. Thinking globally, and acting locally, as the well-worn bumper-sticker proclaims, is key. However, we should also not assume that our mindful consumption is any less an act of consumption, or any more an act of politics or activism, than any other purchase. Mindful consumption is still a form and function of privilege and an example of limited power. And consumption comes back around to the things our body most needs.

Water is a constructive example for considering mindful consumption. Recently, a colleague of mine — a woman in her early 60s with a slew of health problems — discovered the power of water. She would complain often of her many ailments, some of which were interfering with her job, let alone her quality of life. She didn't drink water. When she told me that she started drinking water and that many of her problems were getting better, I was shocked. It was not the miracle cure of water that surprised me but the fact that she didn't drink water. She gestured toward the bathroom and said that she didn't want to be in there every hour. Because I drink water almost exclusively, it never even occurred to me that this would have been her problem. And I drink a lot of water. I can't imagine not drinking water and how absolutely non-functional I would be without it.

And yet, to not have any worry about access to water is a privilege. In other places, women's work(out) is found through the long distances travelled to procure water from limited, and widely shared, supplies. They bear the weight of providing for their families as well as the literal weight of the water. In the U.S., we take water for granted, even when we live in states or cities impacted by drought conditions. We consume it in mass quantities — for refining oil, for raising cattle, for watering our lawns (and golf courses), and for filling our swimming pools (and fountains). Like so many other things, we don't pay attention to where it comes from, and we assume it will be there when we need it. And, yet, we consume other beverages in masse: coffee of every variety and variation, soft drinks, sports drinks, bottled water, and nutritional supplements. And beer and wine and hard alcohol and "light" versions of all of these. We forget the power of water even as it nourishes our own bodies.

Water literally nourishes our bodies and minds; figuratively, water comes with the weight of the world attached. To move our mind/body fitness beyond the individual, oppositional consciousness is crucial.

Developing Critical Consciousness

"The body does not experience the world in the way that consciousness does."

— Peggy Phelan, as quoted in "An Elegy
for Dancing" by Christina Pugh (21)

"Outer development can only be measured against inner development. This inner development relates to consciousness ... individuals are sources of mutual inspiration, who may further the development of consciousness among all human beings."

— Rosina-Fawzia Al-Rawi, *Grandmother's Secrets* (152)

When we speak of consciousness in fitness, we are most often referring to one's relationship between her mind and her body, the ability to listen to one's body and connect the mind and body in purposeful, pleasurable, safe, effective fitness movements. Feminism, as a perspective or philosophy, builds consciousness. Yoga, as a spiritual practice (or fitness practice, we might argue), can build consciousness. Both have their limitations and possibilities. Consciousness is a term that can encompass a variety of meanings and applications; it can also be a complicated and misunderstood term. For instance, consciousness is not the same as conscience, though conscience and conscious can *sound* very similar. Consciousness is not simply the voice nagging the back of the mind. For instance, Alisa Valdés demonstrates her feminist consciousness in her "Ruminations of a Feminist Fitness Instructor," but when it comes down to it, it is problems of *conscience*, not consciousness that causes her to leave the world of fitness. She writes, "I betrayed myself, betrayed my dreams; most of all I betrayed my gender.... I had been duped into believing there was strength in, well, fat loss. Eventually, my conscience got the better of me" (28). She feels guilty about what she sees as misguided attempts to develop a feminist theory of the fitness she is promoting. If she were to employ *consciousness*, unfettered by conscience, she might have felt differently about the work she was doing. She might have found a way to merge her dreams of being a feminist writer with her practical work as a fitness instructor. She might have found a way to work to transform that which she did not like in the fitness industry.

Consciousness is always developing and adapting as we learn; it is a flexible aspect of our minds. Critical consciousness requires us to look beyond the easy answers, to be what bell hooks calls an "enlightened witness"; as such "we are able to be critically vigilant about both what is being told to us and how we respond to what is being told" (*Cultural Criticism*). If we can be "critically vigilant" in the ways in which we observe and understand fitness (mis)-representations, as well as the ways in which we respond to these representations, then there is potential to create change. But growing consciousness in fitness does not simply mean a better relationship with our body. It does not simply mean that we feel movement, create power, or ease into transitions. This is part of the work of fitness. But the deeper work of consciousness is an opening of the mind, a shifting of perspective, a connection outside of one's self. Tara Brabazon explains how we might begin to use fitness toward developing consciousness. She writes, "fitness, exercise and diet can and should be used as a site of consciousness, a pivotal moment where women realize that the consumerist culture has not created a socially just smorgasbord.... We can learn strength by encouraging physical movement, coordination and fitness" (76). Such discoveries and developments of consciousness — on the individual and structural level — cannot be made alone; we need to arm ourselves with ideas and practical tools.

Development of consciousness beyond the individual, the personal, the introspective, requires further connection and development through education and exploration beyond individual, literal, or ephemeral considerations. As a tool of survival and critique of oppression, in the early 1900s, W.E.B. DuBois developed the idea of double consciousness — a "sense of always looking at one's self through the eyes of others" (2) — in his foundational work *The Souls of Black Folk*.[7] He explains that he lives in "a world which yields him no true self-consciousness, but only lets him see himself through the revelation of the other world" (2). This version of consciousness can remind us that there is a set of demands that we might feel we need to live up to, a set of rules created by what bell hooks terms white supremacist capitalist patriarchy. Just as double consciousness helps black people negotiate how to live by one set of expectations in white society and another in black society, this concept might also help us to recognize the constructed nature of the expectations in both these spaces. Likewise, for those oppressed by confining structures, a personal understanding of fitness is shadowed by "the other world."

As feminism gained influence in the 1950s, 60s, and 70s, consciousness-raising groups were important tools. Many great thinkers have shared the responsibility of feminist consciousness-raising on the local, national, and global levels, within and across difference. Individuals were able to see the bigger picture of their experience. The individual struggles of women were, in fact, not isolated, but connected as a part of a larger pattern of patriarchy, a pattern reinforced by white supremacy, capitalism, and heteronormativity. In turn, these oppressive structures create a type of consciousness understood as "oppositional consciousness," a way of seeing the world that recognizes, and works to correct, injustice of all kinds. In "Social Movements and Oppositional Consciousness," from *The Making of Oppositional Consciousness*, Morris and Braine describe oppositional consciousness, in short, as: "an empowering mental state that prepares members of an oppressed group to act to undermine, reform, or overthrow a system of human domination" (25).

Differential consciousness, a form of oppositional consciousness, also has a necessary flexibility; it "operates as process and shifting location" (Sandoval 139), much like the fitness metaphor of flexibility. (It is also like María Lugones' "'world'-travelling.") This theory is developed and explained (in highly theoretical jargon and through complex theoretical foundations) by Chela Sandoval; it is a part of the "methodology of the oppressed." This kind of consciousness is built from oppression and navigates toward social change; it also speaks to the creative and critical approaches explored in *Women and Fitness in American Culture*. "To deploy a differential oppositional consciousness," Sandoval argues, "one can depend on no (traditional) mode of belief in one's own subject position or ideology"; however, these modes will be "called up and utilized ... to act in an also (now obviously) constituted social world" (3). In other words, as we navigate through different situations, our previous experiences inform our movements, even as we search for a new frame of reference, a new way to move through the spaces we inhabit. Later, Sandoval further explains "differential consciousness"; she writes:

> Differential consciousness is linked to whatever is not expressible through words. It is accessed through poetic modes of expression: gestures, music, images, sounds, words that plummet or rise to ... claim their due. This mode of consciousness ... functions outside speech, outside academic criticism, in spite of all attempts to pursue and identify its place of origin [140].

While fitness is not immediately recognizable as differential consciousness, movement is often "not expressible through words" and the arts of fitness are certainly a "poetic mode of expression" that combines "gestures, music, images, sounds, and words." So, if movement specifically, and fitness more generally, share potential for oppositional and differential consciousness, then there is potential for transformation in and through fitness (which is outside speech and academic criticism). Fitness as a "mode of consciousness" can provide tools, what Jane Mansbridge calls "ideational resources — ideas available in the culture that can be built upon to create legitimacy, a perception of injustice, righteous anger, solidarity, and a belief in the group's power" (7). Understanding mainstream fitness constructs and representations through this lens might help to build "emotional involvement" (7) that goes beyond the individual's relationship to fitness.

Because oppositional consciousness also requires "institutional resources" (7), connections must be made across barriers of class, gender, race, and sexuality. Further, the ways in which individuals and groups navigate "required cultural materials" is a blueprint for critical transformations. Mansbridge continues:

> The cultural materials required come in sedimented layers. Individuals in the subordinate group must be *brought together by existing or developing institutions* in order to help one another *dig into those layers, recognize, borrow, modify, inflect, and selectively inflate and suppress* elements from the existing culture to craft what then become new ideas [7, my emphasis].

In theory, at least, recognizing the problems with mainstream versions of fitness, coming together with others who are also concerned with these problems, employing institutional resources, and creating ideational resources are some of the first steps in a long process of critical transformation and development of new ideas. Oppositional consciousness is key, and mind/body fitness methods coalesce with oppositional consciousness as we "dig into those layers" and transform the existing culture.

All of these academic theories of consciousness go much deeper and get much more complicated and nuanced, what's important here is to recognize the importance of other ways of seeing, other ways of knowing, other ways of doing. Today, fitness consciousness continues to be dominated by the same systems of inequality that create and extend oppression amongst "the oppressed." In *21st Century Yoga*, Carol Horton reminds us that "it's critical to be as conscious as possible about how yoga is being culturally represented, pedagogically communicated, and collectively experienced" (xii). The more we consider how we might promote consciousness through movement, the more potentially powerful fitness can become. Perhaps the "99%" is oppressed … until we exercise our ability to see beyond the surface and move deeper, developing critical consciousness.[8]

* * *

Fitness consciousness is a process that involves the physical, emotional, ideological, social, and kinesthetic. Mind/body transformations are certainly linked to a developing critical consciousness. As Paula Lökman explains, "the learning of Aikido techniques changed the ways the women of the study related to their bodies and, as a result, to everyday realities … a new kind of body consciousness emerged" (277). The movements and practice of Aikido, like other fitness forms, has the ability to change body consciousness and consciousness of space and movement. When Markula suggests that "we need to teach participants to feel the movement, to find their own rhythm, to find their own bodies" (75), she is speaking to one kind of fitness consciousness, an awareness of movement, a mindful experience.

In the fitness studio (the pool, the roads) consciousness is only sometimes on the agenda. Even people attending mind/body classes like yoga may be there only for the workout. But this also makes fitness spaces potentially ripe for consciousness-raising. People aren't expecting to have their minds opened to other ways of knowing, being, perceiving, and filtering their own or others' experiences. I often work in some kind of consciousness-raising in bits and pieces, whether these pieces come from the philosophies learned in my trainings or from my own experiences and interpretations. The more sources we draw from for inspiration, the more we practice critical consciousness in fitness movement and critiques; the more we share our feminist knowledge and practice, the more potential we create.

The Power of Dance

"Energy moves in waves. Waves move in patterns. Patterns move in rhythms. A human being is just that, energy, waves, patterns, rhythms. Nothing more. Nothing less. A dance."
— Gabrielle Roth, creator of 5 Rhythms

"While I dance I cannot judge, I cannot hate, I cannot separate myself from life. I can only be joyful and whole. That is why I dance."
— Hans Bos quoted in *The Crescent Moon*, 1995

"The formula is simple: submission to the music, allowing it to guide and direct, equals dancing."
— Jorge "Popmaster Fabel" Pabon in *Total Chaos*

"Dance is holy, sexual, and it's a way of being very powerful and a little dangerous without being violent."
— Eve Ensler, One Billion Rising

The most feminist of my forays into fitness consciousness — and the most personally transformative — are those creative/critical creations of fitness dance. As Al-Rawi argues, "Dancing also stimulates the unconscious, which in turn leads to a widened consciousness and an expanded personality" (56). The possible effects of dance are also noted by Harvard scientists and circulated via social media. The fact that dance wards off dementia better than any other forms of physical activity, and even better than puzzles and brain games, was shared with me by a male colleague who observed and photographed some

Organic Dance at the end of a student conference. He is like Hans Bos, quoted above, who wrote his observations of dance not from his own dance experience, but from his observation of other people dancing. Consciousness-raising in academic settings has its own challenges, but intellectual engagement is expected even as public displays of dance might be resisted. Dancing might also transform our mind/body relationships. Al-Rawi continues, "Dancing offers the consciousness and the unconscious, the rational and the intuitive, a space in which they may gradually flow into each other" (57). In theory, if not in practice, dancing is a convergence of mind and body, of consciousness in development.

* * *

I might say that I discovered the power of dance as a child. But that would not be true. What I discovered in dance class as a child was that I did not like to be on stage, and I really did not like to be on stage in the middle of a chaotic mass of kids flopping their arms and legs around. Dance was not about freedom, expression, innovation, exploration or connecting with yourself or others; it was about learning the steps and performing them in the way you were *supposed to* perform them. My mother thought that dance lessons were an important activity (and she had enjoyed dance herself) and, thus, I took ballet and tap and jazz dance as a young child. My short-lived stint as a wannabe dancer in junior high convinced me that I really was not meant to be a dancer. The narrow context of dance kept its power just out of reach. I thought I was incapable of such art and movement.

I turned to sports not because I was particularly good at them, but because my parents required physical/social activities and sports were compulsory. As awkward or as disappointing as my athletic performances might have been, the movement performed was uniform. I was not different; I was not expressing myself. I was only more, or less, skilled than the other players. I secretly continued to love dance, and I watched music videos or the TV Show *FAME*. When the film version of *A Chorus Line* came out my mother took me to see it even though she said I was too young to understand a lot of it. What I did understand was the passion, and the stories the characters told about how they discovered dance, and the diversity of people who are drawn to dance. (Later, I realized what an important connection this movie was, and is, between me and my mother.) I wanted to discover my dance, my passion.

My passion for fitness is not far off; however, I did not rediscover dance until I took belly dancing classes around the age of 30. Even then, I didn't really think about it as dancing, and I really didn't intend to do anything with it. Fitness, like sports, was uniform movement. My dancing stayed in the confines of my kitchen or living room. I practiced the moves using Hip Hop (mostly the Black Eyed Peas, *Behind the Front*) rather than traditional belly dancing music. Hip-hop is what moved my body and helped me to learn these new movements. The music made me want to move. I slowly began to let go of the linear, boxy, hard movements of step and kickboxing, finding flow and the continuous motions of circles and figure eights and control through isolations.

The power of dance began to become more and more apparent the more I danced, and the more I paid attention to dance. It wasn't just frivolous performance — it was movement and expression. The TV show *So You Think You Can Dance* was a part of this. Being able to see all of the different dance styles, to learn a little about these styles, and to see them performed with passion and emotion was a powerful reminder of my own passion. It was a reminder of what dance can mean to people and how it can transform bodies and ideas, personalities and lives. As I began to explore different forms of dance through fitness, like Nia and Group Groove, I began to discover how much I loved to dance. And as I discovered how much I love to dance, I began to explore less structured dance spaces like 5 Rhythms. (Other variations like Shiva Rea's Trance Dance and Danielle Eastman's Kaya Fitness have a similar approach.) I also began to develop my own transformative "brand" of fitness dance and a mind/body feminist philosophy behind what I do in my classes. The incarnations of fitness dance have morphed from "Girls' Night Out" to "Power, Pleasure, and Movement" to "Feminist Fitness" to "Just Dance" to "Organic Dance." Each variation has subtle differences and varying successes; discovering the power of dance has many layers.

* * *

"Dancers who enter the studio to translate choreography into performance begin by learning the movement, its timing, and its disposition for body in space ... meticulously.... Yet they also modify the movement so as to develop a personal relationship with it. ... to 'make it their own,' ...They may elaborate a persona — an integrative conception of the body-subject who would move in the way specified in the choreography — and then use this concept to further refine stylistic features of their performance."
                                                — Al-Rawi, *Grandmother's Secrets* (9)

The power of dance is found in the power of movement and connection. Thus, my interest in dance is not so much in the performative art form as it is in the embodied movement experience; the two are connected. But in fitness settings, sometimes performance is given precedence. During a Zumbathon, watching 13 instructors come up on stage for two songs each, it became very clear that performance is at the heart of Zumba instruction. I showed up to the event in a plain black tank top and brown yoga pants; at the end of the week my favorite workout clothes were in the laundry, but this was a version of my usual. The other instructors were decked out in Zumba gear, bright colors, sexy ripped and cut shirts that revealed their bellies, full-on make-up, and sparkles everywhere. When they "taught" their songs they were beautiful and sexy, animated and athletic. And silent. They had "perfect bodies" and showed them off. Since I rarely take Zumba, and when I do I only take it from instructors I know and like, I was totally unprepared for the show.[9] There was no instruction, no cueing, only performance to a pulsing, pounding beat. I couldn't hear my body; I couldn't feel the movement. After the event my ears were pounding all night and into the next day, and I was nauseous and sore. I lamented the lost connections and communications. While I had hoped to glean some new moves, the night was a jumble of sights and sounds. I retained little. And my body hurt, badly.

* * *

Perhaps the most powerful discovery I have made through dance — the most empowering aspect and the aspect with the most potential power — is the "playful" aspect. This play is counter to the play of sport.[10] This playful aspect is informed by Nia and Group Groove as much as it is by Lugones' description of play:

> The playfulness that gives meaning to our activity include uncertainty, but in this case the uncertainty is an *openness to surprise*. This is a particular metaphysical attitude that does not expect the world to be neatly packaged, ruly.... We are not wedded to a particular way of doing things. While playful we have not abandoned ourselves to, nor are we stuck in, any particular "world." We are there *creatively*. We are not passive [author's emphasis 400].

An aerobics participant who is used to the rigidity of a routine, the familiarity of a pattern, the stability of a mirror image (instructor and reflection), is uncertain or even frightened by an invitation to dance freely. I have been there. Feeling frozen, unsure what to do, afraid to move without direction and without the safety that comes from being surrounded by uniform movement. Free dance is certainly "unruly," but this can become "an *openness to surprise*." When we break out of a structured routine and move as we feel, we might be surprised about where our movement takes us. And because we are "not wedded to a particular way of doing things," we are free to do things in any particular way. This is a philosophy that crosses fitness forms and beyond.

In part two, I described the overlapping methodology of "building a toolbox." Haphazard, fortuitous, semi-conscious fumblings can build a set of tools. Collecting such tools playfully might make these tools more powerful. This playful collection, examination, and re-arrangement is the dance that this book attempts — to present a diverse set of tools for understanding fitness from the individual to structural, personal to political, playful to serious. This playful excursion has intersectional analysis — another kind of dance — as its foundation. Drawing from the work of Patricia Hill Collins, Dill and Zambrana explain that "transformative is perhaps one of the best words to characterize this scholarship [intersectional analysis] because it is seen not only as transforming knowledge but using knowledge to transform society" (13).[11] This transformative power speaks to the link between individual and communal approaches to fitness. It speaks to the many examples that I have offered throughout this book — a diverse mix of voices that bring marginalized lived experiences into the conversation, a connection between the individual and the community and the personal structural, and a link between research and practice. A holistic picture of American fitness is akin to a holistic approach to social justice and social change. I offer these sketches, arguments, citations, experiences, and meditations playfully. They are a kind of dance, a weaving and winding. The power of dance is like the power of intersections; both open possibilities and redefine limits.

* * *

We might imply from Lugones that because we "have not abandoned ourselves" our play is a means of self discovery, a means toward empowerment and transformation. And since we are there "*creatively*" and we are "not passive," our self exploration is a part of a bigger picture. The connection between our selves and our worlds might be one of the most powerful aspects of dance that we are only beginning to discover. When we dance we can experience self-construction, flexibility, defiance of limiting structures, creativity, consciousness, freedom, and community. This is some of the power of dance that Eve Ensler attempts to tap into in her vision of One Billion Rising, an action/demonstration/movement that asks women and their allies to "Strike Dance Rise!" to gather, take up public space, and dance in order to raise awareness about, and inspire action toward, an end to violence against women. On the "Why We Rise" section of the website, One Billion Rising is described as:

A global strike, an invitation to dance, a call to men and women to refuse to participate in the status quo until rape and rape culture ends, an act of solidarity demonstrating to women the commonality of their struggles and their power in numbers, a refusal to accept violence against women and girls as a given, a new time and a new way of being.

One billion is the estimated number of women around the world who will be raped or beaten in their lifetime and "one billion women dancing is a revolution."[12]

Part of the power of this movement is its adaptability across place and context. This event is serious, but it is also flexible and playful. The Frequently Asked Questions section of the website offers support as well as freedom. "We want you to make One Billion Rising (OBR) your own. Be creative, get wild, connect with other activists and create the event that you imagine. There is no list of strict rules to follow: we want you to fully embrace your leadership!" As a result, groups and organizations, instructors and studios, writers and artists, workers and thinkers, politicians and activists, and college campuses and communities (in more than 200 countries) created events to participate in One Billion Rising. After the event on February 14, 2013 (the 15th anniversary of V-Day), the onebillionrising.org website included video evidence of such risings as far and wide as San Francisco, New York, Kolkata and many other cities in India, São Paulo (Brazil), Manila (Philippines), New Zealand, Khartoum (Sudan), Jerusalem, Chicago, Philadelphia, Ohio, Atlanta, South Africa, and more. Photos and videos were also shared in other social media spaces like Facebook and Twitter. Events ranged from the big screen outside the Los Angeles Staples Center to local venues with an iPod and a speaker. Many of these gatherings used the song "Break the Chain" which was produced specifically for this project (written and produced by Tena Clark) and is featured on the site as a YouTube video.

On the website there are also a number of other videos including a short film about a spectrum of violence against women, "One Billion Rising," and an illustration of the power of women who rise together to end such violence. Scenes of abuse turn to the raising of fists with one finger extended and scenes of women dancing across cultures and contexts. There are also videos to learn the choreography created by Debbie Allen, including an instruction video produced by the Senior dance class at the Brooklyn High School of the Arts. In some spaces, celebrity endorsement dominates. In other spaces the everyday practice of dance is transformed into part of a bigger movement.

Ensler's words and inspiration help to support and promote the movement and even speak to the importance of men's support for this event through the video created by Tony Stroebel, "Man Prayer." In this video Ensler's words are brought to life as a variety of men and boys deliver lines from this piece in a variety of languages and the words in English are displayed on the screen. Personal messages from Ensler also provide support and inspiration. One week before One Billion Rising, "A Message from Eve" YouTube video on the website urges us to think about why dance is important:

> I think most of us women ... we don't move the way we want because we're afraid on some level of being attacked ... the whole idea is that we break out of this cage of patriarchy, of fear and intimidation, and we blast open the boundaries that have kept our selves, kept our creativity, kept our body in prison. And we discover this new energy which is going to fuel the planet and make ... all the things that matter to us possible. Let's make February 14th the biggest, massive, most joyous, fiercest action the world has ever known.

Ensler makes connections between the individual act of dancing and the overcoming of fear and the challenging of the system of patriarchy that has "kept our body in prison." She also thanks everyone for believing in dance and for bringing their communities together. Perhaps it is a stretch to jump from this empowerment to a "new energy" that can transform "all the things that matter to us." Or perhaps this is exactly the stretch that such movement makes possible. My students make me think so. After a long day at an interdisciplinary conference, I'm thinking that no one is going to want to do the planned closing activity — Organic Dance. As the presentations wind down, my students made the decision that not only were we going to dance, we were going to dance *outside*. It was a perfect afternoon in Maine, a rarity in April. Because it was Friday, the campus was virtually empty. We danced in the grass, through the wind, under the moving clouds. We danced despite the photographer and seated observer. We moved. We went from run-down to rejuvinated.

Cynical or hopeful, or somewhere in between, the power of dance is clearly something we are only beginning to discover.

Community and Transformative Fitness on the Ground

> "Women need to reach out, find a network, and build a community through spirit, mind, and body. I view this kind of sisterly community building as one of my greatest contributions to feminism...."
> — Wendy Walter-Bailey, "If These Roads Could Talk:
> Life as a Woman on the Run" (148)

> "Can we really expect yogis to run soup kitchens while we're still making our rent? ... It may be another generation before the patina of real

community starts to glow.... I'd like to see us stop *talking* about community, and start actually *doing* community."
— Matthew Remski, "Modern Yoga Will Not Form
a Real Culture...." (112; original emphasis)

While I have explored many variations of transformative fitness, there is no doubt that community can enhance our endeavors both to be more fit and to build more fitness. When we make a commitment to fitness, we make a commitment not just to ourselves but we also make a commitment to community — in literal and figurative forms. Even the most solitary of exercises and the most separatist of routines, is linked to a fitness community. The solitary runner finds that she improves her running when she joins a community and discovers a variety of benefits to having this community. A swimmer shares the pool, often amid lap swimmers, children's splashing, and aqua aerobics. In the weight room, spotters are often required (and are sometimes strangers) and pairs of lifters chat endlessly between and during sets. And in the group fitness room, bodies move in unison, or slightly off-kilter, sharing space and movements, following and finding inner strength. Within any of these micro communities is an endless variation of connection. The bond between the personal trainer and client may be tight while the swimmer may swim to feel alone and buoyant. The person in Zumba may or may not talk to anyone, but she is noticed if only as a part of a whole. We may choose our fitness community or find one by default but it is always there, ready to catch us if we let it. If we work to weave fitness into our communities, the net is even stronger.

Those of us with skills, knowledge, and talents might offer free workshops, donate our time to teach a community class, or take time to talk to a group of cancer survivors about stretching. Local incarnations sprinkle my small campus. Noontime walks, Zumbathon fundraisers, and a Wellness committee are a few examples of fitness community activities. In *21st Century Yoga* Remski suggests what studios can do to provide community like providing a "yoga-based after-school care program" (124) or including a soup kitchen (122).[13] All of these actions build community through a sharing of fitness. Creating a *feminist* community through fitness is not an easy feat, but many of the pieces — like process, shared experience, and well-being — are already in place in gyms, community centers, college recreation centers, fitness centers, neighborhood trails, etc. Communities shift and must be made and remade; such community work is another aspect of fitness-related work. And key to feminist mind/body fitness.

* * *

Because education shapes many of my communities, some of my endeavors to bring fitness into my community stay close to home. For instance, during the fall 2012 semester, one of my colleagues who teaches in our Vet Tech program wanted to reinforce the importance of fitness in her students' lives and in their chosen career path. Caring for animals takes emotional strength in addition to the more obvious physical strength needed to lug 50-pound bags of dog food or to restrain a 150-pound dog. As a part of her initiative she engaged students in a variety of activities including lugging bags of food, attending a weight room orientation, and listening to guest speakers. I visited her class and shared with them my experience and knowledge, focusing on the ideas of "functional" and "mindful" fitness. She was hoping to build a community of students committed to fitness, who would better serve their clients (animals) and who would better serve themselves by staying healthy and fit, ready for life's inevitable challenges.

Sometimes we have to sneak fitness information into our classes, and other times we are fortunate to have a space where such information is the very reason for being in class. In the fall of 2012 I offered a new course at my university, a part of both the American Studies and Women's Studies minors and an upper-level elective course for interested students. This course was offered as a hybrid class; I had two groups of students — one on each campus — and each group alternated between live class meetings with me and online work. In a class with about 30 students, about half the students had no prior experience with American Studies or Women's Studies.

Teaching this new, experimental course, I could not have asked for a better group of students. They took on their work with earnestness and often enthusiasm. While a few students dropped and few missed two or three classes, the vast majority of students didn't miss any classes — live and online. The class was composed of about 30 students (in two locations) and about equal numbers of men and women, which is unusual for my campus, whose student population is about 70 percent female. Students' ages ranged from early twenties through to a student in his sixties. We had a tentative start, getting used to the hybrid format, but once students discovered the flexibility and the direct, personal relevance of the material, they produced excellent, thoughtful, engaged work. The two sites operated differently and had different kinds of conversations, and students brought, and took with them, different experiences and perspectives on fitness. As a community this allowed us to explore diverse interests and aspects of fitness.

Throughout this course, students learned to consider "fitness" as a far more complicated concept and as a concept that held individual as well as social and cultural importance. Students' assignments included creating Wiki entries for fitness products and experiences and completing a personal fitness project as well as an action/education project. All of their work was a joy to read. The Personal Fitness Project was my favorite as students attempted a personal fitness intervention or experiment particular to their needs and interests — quitting smoking, starting juicing, cutting out soda, trying yoga, walking. Their reflections embraced the assignment. They celebrated successes and lamented challenges, but each was honest and unique and contextualized their personal experiences through ideas from class.

Students' final work in this course covered a broad array of topics from the personal to the political, the individual to the structural. Some did more traditional research-based projects while others created community resources or recreation spaces. Some topics of projects included: misrepresentations of women in sports, the healing powers of yoga, longevity, running, pregnancy and fitness (done by a male student), and representations of fitness and fitness messages on television. Two of the more advanced papers included an individual and structural analysis of transformation (including psycho-social barriers to exercise) which was also a beginning framework for an interdisciplinary capstone in Art Therapy. Another advanced paper explored the "underlying trends that cause disparities in American health and community." More action-oriented projects included reviving a community/school hiking/snow shoeing trail, creating a website with information about local area walking trails (accompanied by an excellent analysis of the healing powers of walking and running), a campus-event presentation about raising rabbits for meat (nutritious and renewable), and a creation of a fitness program for an academic summer youth program. This diversity of projects was a result of a flexible, intersectional pedagogy that allows students to find their own way within a larger framework of material and approaches. The methods in my academic classes embrace the fitness method and metaphor of flexibility.

My students in American studies and women's studies often note how much they wished they had learned "this stuff" before college. In addition to my regular fitness teaching in the community, I have looked for ways to bring transformative ideas about fitness to youth. A barrier to youth-related fitness programs is underscored by one of the most important reasons we need such programs — youth are not encouraged to think about fitness. Programs that emphasize movement, or play, or a healthy diet are offering a part of the bigger picture of physical fitness. Perhaps there is more potential in programs that emphasize a mind-body approach and a bigger picture of the meaning and purpose of movement. There are certainly many incarnations of this phenomenon. With more attention to particular methods and materials that can help to augment a mind-body fitness mode, there is the potential to transform young people's relationship to fitness before it is fully developed. More particularly, before it is fully developed as defined by the mold of "American fitness."

I have begun to develop such programs for middle school and high school students and hope to grow them more in the future. In the summer of 2009, I participated in Cougar Quest, a summer program at Washington State University that brings junior high students one week and high school students the next week to live in the dorms and attend classes. I offered a class, "Culture and Fitness: Yoga, Belly Dancing, and Hip Hop," that met for four days, about two hours a day. We started with definitions of fitness, and the students created collages to represent what they saw as "fitness." We discussed and practiced these forms of fitness and concluded by discussing what we had learned. I was surprised at how successful this workshop was overall. It got positive feedback on the students' evaluations and from my observations of the students' work. I tried a version of this workshop as a month-long series at the Camden Teen Center in Maine the following fall. This endeavor was a massive failure. The teen center is an almost completely unstructured environment, and the workshop was advertised on a flier on the bulletin board. As long as students are following their basic rules (mostly etiquette and safety) they can do pretty much what they like including a vast array of video games, TV, homework, a skate park, and other activities. My workshop was only one of many choices and was not advertised outside of the normal population that frequents the center, mostly 5th to 7th grade. From this success and failure, I fashioned another workshop for students at the high school level.

The most successful workshop I have offered was called "Getting College Fit," a name that I did not choose but which became inconsequential. It was a required afternoon activity in the YoUMA program during the summer of 2011, a day camp at the University of Maine at Augusta that allows students to earn one college credit, taking a class in the morning and attending other activities in the afternoon. Other afternoon activities included a museum trip, service at a local homeless shelter, and a swimming excursion at a local park. (During this day camp I also taught a highly successful academic class about media representations and popular culture to five girls.) This workshop offered students a bigger picture of what physical and mental "fitness" might mean to a college student.

The group of students I had at the afternoon fitness workshop was pretty evenly split between boys and girls and, during discussion, almost all of the students participated with enthusiasm. We began by talking about what "fitness" is and how we might define it. I shared a few interesting facts with them like the definitions of fitness from the AMA and ACE. I also shared with them the invention of the term aerobics by Kenneth Cooper and the significance of the year 1968. We talked about how we might see strength, flexibility, balance, and endurance as metaphors as well as physical states. I also told them about my personal and professional fitness experience, especially as it pertained to college.

After this brief discussion we split into several groups. Some of my students volunteered to help me with the workshop. One student took a group out to play soccer, another took a group to walk on the fitness trails, and the third group stayed with me to do belly dancing. The group who stayed to do belly dancing were two girls, both members of the Somali Muslim population that has grown in Maine. The soccer group was the biggest group, and a handful of students went on the walking trails. I wanted to be sure that the students had a choice of fitness activities so that they could choose the one they were most comfortable with. I expected that only a few students would select the belly dance activity; it is best as a self-selected activity. Two of my students joined the girls from the YoUMA program and we shared belly dance movement in a moment of expression and connection.

After we did our activities of choice, we came back and discussed the activities, reflecting back upon our earlier discussion about fitness. We talked about what they did, how they felt they were experiencing those aspects of fitness, what made each activity different and how they were similar. The students discussed their activities voraciously and had many insights about the differences and similarities, benefits and potential of these activities. The belly dance students were more reserved in their sharing, as I expected, but they still made important contributions to our conversation and the joy and confidence they gained through the activity was clear.

We ended the workshop by getting in a circle and doing some basic yoga postures. There were some giggles and general discomforts, but, generally, the students participated in the yoga exercises with some seriousness. I chose poses that were easy, yet challenging, so that they would be successful but also interested in learning more. We did some warriors poses, tree pose balance, down dog and prayer position, and seated stretches. We ended in a few minutes of final relaxation. While this workshop was just a small taste of fitness, I was surprised at how well the students responded to it. I expected far more students to not want to participate or to not take it seriously, but they engaged with all of the aspects of the workshop with some enthusiasm. Both of these workshops illustrate how important exposure to ideas about fitness are for youth to develop positive relationships with their active bodies — as well as the potential to transform dominant, narrow ideas about fitness.

The potential for further development of youth-oriented fitness programs that focus on the mind and body, the critical and creative, and pleasure and process, is ripe. Similar programs for other groups might begin to bring us all face to face with the potential of feminist mind/body fitness.

New Connections: Teaching Facing

> "Aerobics ... holds a pedagogical function, teaching corporeal literacies, physical coordination, balance and also intricate and complicated affiliations between individual goals and desires, and those of the group."
> "When aerobics participants turn to face the mirror, myriad ambiguous, if not contradictory, gazes are reflected back. The critical eye — that compares, critiques and attacks the self — is concurrently paired with the challenging 'I' of empowerment, community and fitness."
> — Tara Brabazon, "Fitness Is a Feminist Issue" (79; 68)

From the very beginning of my fitness teaching I was trained to face away from the class, facing front, toward the mirrors, my back to the class. This orientation allows participants to follow your body position and footwork, and they can look in the mirror to see what you/they are doing. You step with your right foot, they step with their right foot. You lift your left arm, they lift their left arm. This is the easy way to follow. When I had taken classes with instructors facing the participants (which was rare), I would often get sides and directions confused. I'm already left/right and spatially challenged. The instructor's movement did not make sense as my opposite. I struggled with the need to teach facing when participating in a Zumbathon, on a stage in a gym, with no mirrors. I did not think it was possible. When I practiced I felt awkward. I didn't know if I could do it. And then the event happened and I just did it. Facing the people made sense. There was nowhere else to look. When I moved to Bangor, I joined a group of instructors who, for the most part, teach facing. I dove in and tried this new teaching style.

Teaching facing requires one to say left when she steps right and right when she moves left. Step is more confusing and facing the instructor requires different spacial reasoning. It was difficult to learn how to take classes with the instructor facing us. Dance moves are more difficult, belly dancing moves especially, as circular movements are difficult to gage when looking at a mirror image. But taking classes from this orientation certainly made it easier to learn to teach facing the class. In fact, after taking my favorite class — Group Groove — for a while I found myself desiring to begin on the left instead of the right, to turn around and face the opposite direction, to be on the instructor's side. And now teaching facing is the direction I teach from in all of my classes.

To teach facing requires eye contact and personal engagement. It requires that an instructor be aware of the participants' reactions. Eye contact and awareness can both be achieved with the mirrors when facing away; but to teach facing also requires an instructor to be adept, to move opposite to the way that the entire class is moving, to communicate her movements in a way that is still clear despite the lack of a direct, similarly-oriented movement model. Teaching facing requires a kind of disconnect from one's own body/image. We cannot see ourselves as a model for our own movement; we have to trust that what we feel is also the model we are providing. We have to have body awareness.

I still sometimes teach facing away, facing the mirror, most often upon request from students or when teaching complicated step patterns. I've also found greater success facing away in Cardio Kickboxing. But teaching facing the participants is more natural to me now, and this mode meshes with feminist fitness. Teaching facing requires a connection with students that is not always easy to make when connecting through a mirror surface. Teaching facing opens the instructor, rather than closing her away. Her presence is real and immediate and not mediated. She is the mirror.

Mind/Body Empowerment, Flexibility and Pleasure

Intuitive Eating Principle #6: "Discover the Satisfaction Factor."[14]

"I think the empowering really comes from again that getting more in touch with who you are ... it's very simple. You can be yourself versus trying to be something else."
— Elise Browning Miller, Iyengar yoga teacher and founding director of California Yoga Center, quoted in *Yoga Is*

"If participants in group exercise classes are encouraged to think more about the sensuous pleasure during exercise, gyms and health clubs might enjoy greater member retention ... if the fitness industry could adopt a more playful — a word I use quite intentionally — attitude toward exercise, participants might begin to understand their moving bodies in completely different ways. Not only might this transform thinking of exercise as a necessary task (or even as drudgery) but could decrease exercise-related injuries and possibly reduce stress levels further."
— Pirkko Markula, "It's Fun When It's Over," from *Psychology Today* blog

Gina Kolata ends her book about "ultimate fitness" by noting the importance of pleasure. Markula's research shows the importance of pleasure. I base my personal fitness routine and the classes I choose to teach on pleasure. Pleasure in movement, strength, community, or whatever fitness benefits we need and value, is a key aspect to mind/body empowerment through fitness. This pleasure should not be confused with luxury. "Poetry is not a luxury," as feminist poet and critic Audre Lorde reminds us in *Sister Outsider*. Neither is fitness. The basic concepts of fitness, strength, flexibility, balance, and agility have deeper meanings than their physiological measurements. As metaphors, they are tools for negotiation. The more we think about these metaphors, the more relevance fitness has to our lives, our daily struggles of all kinds. This relevance is most realized with attention to mind and body in tandem. The more we move consciously, the more we'll be consciously moved.

Feminists and researchers have found *both* empowerment *and* disempowerment in women's experiences in aerobics classes. This gendered activity is considered to play too much to stereotypes of femininity; likewise, it is considered to be "a disempowering technique of bodily discipline that mainly reinforces the oppressive physical ideal" (Kennedy and Markula 9). This disempowering quality is directly linked to the kind of atmosphere that aerobics provides as well as the attitude of fitness professionals in these spaces. Kennedy and Markula argue that such research results have caused critical feminist researchers to turn to other kinds of exercise that might not reinforce feminine ideals, like bodybuilding or weight lifting (10). As feminist researchers reconsider a variety of fitness spaces, the contradictions will remain as long as the dominant idea of American fitness is focused on appearance and gendered stereotypes. As Kennedy and Markula note, Debra Gimlin has argued that "aerobics can serve as cultural resource for alternative constructions of female beauty" (7). She also discovered that "'working out' made women feel better even without visible change" (8) and this act was "a personally liberating, strong and active choice" (8). When we work to infuse aerobics with critical feminism, we bring the mind to play with the body. We can inspire feminist mind/body fitness that can lead to empowerment and pleasure and all kinds of transformations.

The well-worn metaphor of "wearing many hats" is often used in instructor trainings to teach us how to be empowered in our persona as a fitness instructor. We should not adopt a fake character; we should consider ourselves as instructors as a version of our self— one version among many. The idea of adopting a fitness instructor persona was one of the things that made me weary of becoming a fitness instructor. I knew that there was no way that I could put on a fake, plastic smile. I knew I would never be a picture of perfection. But as Christina Pugh learned in her elegy, "energy is something one can assume and, indeed, something one owes to one's students" (28). And so even with my seriousness, my love shines through, as I find ways to bring energy — and most importantly, joy — into group movement. My fitness persona requires diligence and rejuvenation; and it provides empowerment and pleasure. If we go to the gym or fitness studio for pleasure, in addition to or even instead of the other reasons we go, we have transformed our way of thinking about exercise. We need to have better access to tools toward both empowerment and pleasure if we want to transform ourselves and the ways in which we use and understand fitness. In *Teaching to Transgress*, bell hooks writes of theory, and "reflection and analysis," as healing and liberatory (59–61); the theory of feminist fitness is also such a tool. Armed with feminist fitness, flexibility is key.

Fitness requires a link, or many different kinds of links, between the mind and body. Such linking cannot be rigid or proscribed; it must be fluid and flexible. As Christina Brown argues "physical postures also increase the flow of subtle energies. As you free up the body, you free up the mind. Flexibility in the body promotes mental flexibility, and this brings a sense of ease to life." We all can find our own fitness factors that balance mind and body, and this balance is an important component in and out of the pursuit of fitness. But mental flexibility is more than "a sense of ease" — it is a tool toward transformation.

"'World-travelling,' for Lugones, describes "a particular feature of the outsiders existence: the acquired flexibility in shifting from the mainstream construction of life to other constructions of life where she is more or less 'at home'" (390). While this is a presumed condition for women of color, Lugones notes that "this flexibility is necessary for the outsider but it can also be willfully exercised by those who are at ease in the mainstream" (390). Mainstream expectations of fitness limit our movements and approaches; they apply a "one-size-fits-all" approach despite the evidence to the contrary. There is no one way to be fit just as there is no one way to be a woman, despite what dominant ideas disseminate. While we might not be able to choose the circumstances, we can certainly choose our approach, our place, our way of dealing with and even transforming these circumstances if they are unfit, unjust. The ability to be creative in our existence as well as our arts is an empowering state and can be a way to connect across cultures, across difference. Wearing many hats means not only adopting and adapting personalities or shifting to find "home," it also speaks to a playful way of being.

There are some flexible, playful, pleasure-seeking foundations in fitness space. Gabrielle Roth writes about how we get too attached to our identities, that we should really be comfortable being "everything and nothing" at the same time and 5 Rhythms and Nia encourage us to move and play in a variety of personalities that are less proscribed than a program like Group Groove or Zumba. Flexibility allows us to adapt to adverse conditions and to have several shifting approaches. Flexibility, Michael Stone argues, is something that Patanjali teaches "over and over" (154).[15] But flexibility must be adapted to American consciousness. Stone gives us one theory: "what causes suffering is holding on to inflexible views" (154). While a sacred yoga truth, this truth can be used as a version of blaming the victim since corrupt power and inadequate social support systems (supported by inflexible views) are what cause suffering. Inflexible views are a privilege. Those of us who navigate mainstream constructions and movements that only marginally include us, must be flexible in order to avoid being swept up or crushed. Fortunately, Stone argues, "the same psychological tools that yogis have mapped for helping us let go of one-track rigid stories can be applied not just personally, but socially" (155). The stories we tell ourselves about fitness keep us locked into limited ideas and ideals, individually and collectively. In these circumstances, flexibility — of identity or tactic — is potentially a revolutionary tool. Stone even connects this back to the pleasure "humans are always trying to gain" (155). I have tried to show how we are already imagining different fitness ideas and ideals, and how we might move away from fitness as an individual pursuit and toward fitness as a collective movement.

Too often pursuits of empowerment are confused with those of self-help; this configuration follows our emphasis on the individual as a site of change. For instance, as I, and many others have argued, the mantra of "girl power" is confused with empowerment and girls and women are led to believe that our power comes from our purchase power or our "pussy power" rather than from a strong sense of self and a commitment to our community. Our checkbooks and our bodies are the tools we are given permission to use. Citing the work of Susan Benson who also points out the problems with "good body/bad body" narratives, Brabazon argues, "Benson realises [sic] that when the self becomes a focus and a project there must be a cost to community-based strategies of political resistance, such as feminism" (68). Feminism is also discounted as being, for instance, the reason why we have so many cultural, social, and economic problems, as we saw in the discussion around the idea that "feminism makes you fat." This dual attack on feminism means that both individuals and communities suffer; transformation of self must be seen as more than self-help.

Brabazon worries "that aerobics, fitness and diet have been compliantly slotted into the categories of self-help. Already," she argues, "feminist books are placed on the bookshelves of personal development" (76). Remski makes a similar argument about yoga; this self-help approach "shortsells the real potential of the yoga studio to rise into its role as community center" (123). If we keep these collective issues on the self-help shelf, we miss the opportunity to create structural change — a different role for fitness and new opportunities for community. The biggest problem with the self-help dimension, Brabazon argues, is that "self help, as a genre, rarely recognises [sic] repressive social structures or collective solutions" (76). Many girls and women are led to believe that the problem lies within them rather than within the culture they are a part of. This is one reason why feminism is so important. "The self-help movement focuses on the pain, not the context of the pain. Feminism stresses the causes" (78). Feminism also puts "personal" issues into community context, historical context, and cultural context; and it gives us tools toward empowerment that can work on the individual as well as the collective level, if we're willing to put in the work. Ultimately, Brabazon argues, "Aerobics is an intrinsic activity that gains meaning of and for itself" (66). Extended to consider aerobics as fitness more generally, the more we invest in a feminist mind/body fitness regime that feeds empowerment, the more this activity gains meaning and importance in and of itself. And often this meaning is — at its base — pleasure. And this pleasure is much better when we share it.

As I have argued, critical perspective is ultimately key to mind/body empowerment. Our inner critic inhibits our movements and limits our consciousness. Our outer critic demands to *see* the differences and encourages "no pain, no gain" mentalities. When we move, we are more open. When we move and feel and find pleasure, we are more likely to embrace change and shift our perspective. When we are flexible in our perspectives, we make more room for other ways of seeing, doing, being. One of the beauties of feminist mind/body fitness is that each of us, both independently and interconnected, can find the particular version of fitness that feeds our souls, bodies, minds, and hearts — an evolving, perhaps lifetime, process and lived practice. These are always also shared; we can transform the unconscious sharing by making it conscious, visible, purposeful. And the beat remains steady, consistent. The movements change us.

Perspective

Horizons set at the door
Or in the back of the mind
A limitation without limits
A fall without rise

> We might set horizons
> As goals to achieve
> We might forget that horizons
> Are also setting suns
>
> We may need horizons
> To remind us of change
> As our bodies age
> And we push for new plateaus
>
> We may need horizons
> As safe points to gaze upon
> As our bodies gage
> Distance and time
>
> Horizons don't move
> Body or mind
> They are always in relation
> In perspective
>
> They are always still waiting
> To be transformed
> By Movement.

The Cool Down (Some Conclusions)

"Transformation. It's an Inside job." — YogaFit t-shirt slogan

"For those of us fortunate enough to live in able bodies we can take to the gym, and for those of us fortunate enough that we don't have to spend every minute of our days scraping for basic survival needs or struggling against overt oppression, life is full of choices. Life is also a series of interruptions.... The one relationship we have that isn't interrupted, at least until the day it permanently ends, is the one we have with our bodies. The most intimate connection we have to our time on this planet, our bodies are home to the lives we live, and the lives we live show on them."

— Myrl Coulter, "Gym Interrupted" (108)

Life's interruptions need not impede transformation. People cycle in and out of fitness initiatives, spaces, groups, and classes, even when they've committed time or money. As a life-long process, we start and stop and begin again and again. This book is one such beginning. I have presented one version of American fitness. It asks us to complicate how we think about fitness and how we think about the connections between our mind and our body. It asks us to challenge the limited conceptualizations of fitness that are presented to us and to create alternatives within or without these structures. It asks us to take women's experiences and challenges as the center, to shift the conversation and expectations of what "fitness" means. Is it naive to think that a radical reconsideration of "fitness" could transform the tightly knit structures that undermine individual and collective fitness? Perhaps. But, we Americans love to transform ourselves. We just need to do so on a deeper level, rather than hovering on the surface. As communities rather than individuals.

We need to recognize that true transformation must be collective. Coulter's assumptions about, and definitions of, "interruptions" gloss over the ways in which oppression and survival "show on" our bodies. These marks are signs of "interruption" as well. Our bodies may be "homes to the lives we live" but, for the oppressed, these homes are devalued and the marks of oppression are both deep and superficial, visible and buried. In this environment, interruption is temporary — bodies/minds shift and resume the work at hand. They survive; and "fitness" is illusive. Definitions as well as practices must be transformed.

In each of the sections of this book I have presented tools and insights, experience and analysis. I have built upon mainstream and historical, academic, and popular definitions of fitness, and I have complicated standard definitions and frequent assumptions. I have further complicated a subject that seems simple on the surface but goes deep and wide in its reach. One of my intentions is to spark conversation — personal and collective considerations of fitness that will move us, individually and collectively toward transformations. I have tried to show where we've been, though I have focused more on the moment where we are — toward an understanding of where we want to be. I've moved and rearranged the shifting pieces; I've tried to keep them moving. American fitness may be a story of "history repeat[ing] itself," like Kolata argues in her second chapter; but this cycle can be shaped. Transformation can be shaped.

* * *

I am not perfect. I do not proclaim to have all the answers. Mine is one voice and one body. For almost 15 years my fitness practice was a side job, a hobby, a change of pace, extra income, a mandated time to work out. As fitness has become more of a part of my life, it has also become a more necessary part of my life. It has embedded itself in my brain and body; it has transformed me. And yet, my state of physical fitness fluctuates with stress and the demands of life and work and family and self-preservation, let alone transformation. I still struggle with many of the issues, contradictions, and challenges that I discuss throughout this book. I still fail some of the people closest to me as they struggle with their own fitness and health issues. But one thing I do know is that without fitness — as a way of life, as an aspect of physical activity, as a subject of interest, as a creative outlet — I would not, and could not, be myself. I wouldn't be able to inspire and serve, support and nurture, teach and learn in the ways that I do. All of the benefits I reap on a daily basis — a better night's sleep; more energy and stamina throughout the day; management of neck, shoulder and wrist pain; a confirmation of my worth and abilities; a community with a shared culture; etc. — are sown from (and re-rooted in) fitness. I also know that every day I hear unsolicited testimony from people who take my fitness classes about how much better they feel as a result of yoga or belly dancing or feminist fitness or running a marathon. Transformations of women's bodies and lives are a result of commitment and balance and a shift of consciousness. I witness such transformations, and I can attest to the radical power and potential of fitness in all of our individual and collective lives.

And I am not the only one. This work grows from the work that has preceded it and speaks to the work that still needs to be done. The examples that I provide from my experience happen in similar ways at gyms, studios, universities, fitness centers, recreation centers, public spaces, and other locales around the U.S. and around the world. There is power in these connections across location and my hope is to push the conversation around women, fitness, and transformation in new directions. I have dug through the layers, but there are plenty of aspects of fitness that I have barely touched, skirted around, or scraped the surface.

So, now we have more work(ing out) to do.

Final Relaxation/Rejuvenation

Voices slide in under the door. The lights flicker on, then off. We push ourselves up from the floor. We inhale/yawn. We gather ourselves, replace socks and sweatshirts, roll up our mats. The next class barrels in as we float out. Stacks of steps, weights, towels, frustration and tension, fill the space. They will work (it) out. We will return, continue the process.

* * *

Most yoga classes end with final relaxation (savasana). While any position can be assumed, "corpse pose" is most common. In this pose arms and legs fall out to the sides, palms face up, eyes close. No tension. Only breath. Stillness of body encourages stillness of mind. Rejuvenation is the most basic of transformations.

When I first started taking/teaching yoga, I hated final relaxation. The only place I can really relax is at home, in bed, usually in the last few moments before I fall asleep. (And I rarely have trouble falling asleep.) Besides, why waste my time lying around when there are a million things to do?! I still struggle to make time for this relaxation/release at the end of class and in my own life. I still struggle to turn my mind off. I, like Elizabeth Gilbert, am not the only one. But sometimes I am not so sure that mental stillness and singular mental focus are the only forms of relaxation, let alone enlightenment. My movement — hips and heart — is meditation. My cues are a rhythmic mantra. Only the words, the breath, the movement, the stillness, the sounds, and the community exist. Perhaps stillness is only a pause in perpetual motion. Stillness. A moment. Relaxation is a dance, a rhythm, a beat, a negotiation of space, an exchange between inner and outer. Another moment. We move together, we move ourselves. We are transformed.

Appendix: Fitness Terms, Products and Personalities

ACE. The American Council on Exercise provides training, education, and up-to-date research in the fitness industry as well as certifications.

AMA. The American Medical Association focuses on improving healthcare outcomes, accelerating change in physician education, and ensuring sustainable physician practices.

Atkins. A diet system that involves limited consumption of carbohydrates that gained popularity in 2003 and 2004.

Beachbody. Parent company to many fitness programs sold via infomercial (like Insanity, Body Beast, Brazil Butt Lift, and Les Mills Pump) that market at-home fitness programs, nutritional plans, and nutrition supplements.

Bikram Yoga. A style of "hot yoga," founded and tightly controlled by Bikram Choudhury. Each class is 90 minutes long and includes the same 26 poses and two breathing exercises.

Body Training Systems (BTS). The Step Company. Works directly with clubs and fitness instructors to provide a System of Management, Training, Programming and Marketing as related to fitness. Programs include Group Groove, Group Step, Group Ride, Group Power, Group Cenergy, and more.

Bounce. Associated with Title Nine. This on-line and catalog shopping sells undergarments that celebrate the actual buyer rather than society's expectation of the buyer's body.

Cardio. A generic term that refers to the cardiovascular components of a workout (Kenneth Cooper's *Aerobics* is the same idea). A cardio workout gets the heart beating faster, the blood pumping harder, and is often seen as a fat-burning or calorie-burning workout.

Cardio Dance. A generic term for group fitness classes that are based upon dance moves. The original incarnation was called dance aerobics. Zumba, Jazzercise, Shimmy Pop, Group Groove, and non-branded forms exist.

Cooper, Kenneth. Coined the term "aerobics" in his book by the same name in 1968. Developed Cooper Wellness and a variety of fitness-related programs.

Cross Fit. Developed by Greg and Lauren Glassman. A program that uses minimal equipment, "garage" gym spaces, and functional fitness for boot camp-style motivation.

Curves. A fitness franchise opened by Gary and Diane Heavin in 1992 that specializes in fitness and weight loss for women. The Curves program includes a 30-minute workout combining strength-training, cardio, and stretching. The largest fitness franchise in the world with locations in 90 countries.

5 Rhythms. Created by Gabrielle Roth in the late 1970s. A program of guided dance. After injuring herself, Roth was instructing dance classes while seated and started to observe the various rhythms being danced.

Flirty Girl Fitness. A fitness program that incorporates dance and choreography to deliver a strength and cardio-based workouts.

Fonda, Jane. A fitness guru as well as an actor, writer, and political activist. Fonda is known not only for her films and fitness videos, but also for her controversial politics during the Vietnam War era. Co-founder of the Women's Media Center.

Group Fitness. A generic term used to describe classes that are taught to a group of people ranging in size. A variety of types of exercise can be taught in this group format from step to cardio dance to boot camp to yoga.

Group Groove. A dance-based group fitness program by BTS. "If you can move, you can Groove."

Hip Hop Abs. A program of Beachbody by Shaun T. It combines a dance/workout routine that claims to improve one's abdominal area by employing hip-hop dance moves.

Hipline. Oakland, CA. Founded by sisters Samar and Gabriela Nassar, Hipline is a dance fitness establishment located in Oakland and Berkeley, California, that teaches dance to women while cultivating a sisterhood community. Shimmy Pop is their particular brand of dance-based fitness.

Horton, Tony (P90X). An American personal fitness instructor, best known for his boot camp style P90X home fitness program.

Insanity. A program of Beachbody by Shaun T. Emphasizes its reputation as the toughest workout on DVD.

Jazzercise. A choreographed dance aerobics phenomenon created by Judi Sheppard Missett in 1969. Popular during the 80s and 90s and still taught in the 2010s. Two-time *Dancing with the Stars* champion, Cheryl Burke, was a company spokesperson.

The Masala Bhangra Workout. Created by Sarina Jain who is described as the "Jane Fonda of India." A dance-based aerobic workout program that combines Bollywood dance moves with traditional Bhangra dance steps.

Michaels, Jillian. Best known for her appearances on *The Biggest Loser*, Michaels is a personal trainer, reality show personality, and entrepreneur from Los Angeles, California. Since 2005 she has released more than 15 DVDs that use a blend of strength training techniques including kickboxing, yoga, Pilates, plyometrics, and weight training.

Mills, Les. A retired New Zealand athlete who represented New Zealand at the Olympic Games. After retiring from active competition, Mills became a gym/business owner. His son Philip Mills founded Les Mills International in his name. Les Mills provides team training and group fitness programs like Bodypump, Bodycombat, Bodyattack, Bodystep, Bodyflow, Bodyvive, and more.

The Nia Technique (Nia). A non-impact physical conditioning program based on the concept that movement is a route of personal transformation and self-discovery. It is typically performed barefoot and involves whole-body conditioning and cardiovascular aerobic exercise.

P90X. A home fitness program designed by Tony Horton which uses cardio training, jump training (plyometrics), and the martial art of kenpo (kempo).

Pilates. A mind/body form of exercise developed by Joseph Pilates that emphasizes stretching and strengthening the core. Originally based in therapy for rehabilitation of soldiers, Mat Pilates classes are offered as well as Pilates classes using the Reformer, a piece of equipment specially designed for Pilates exercises. Pilates also has a variety of props, styles, and a split between modern and classic.

Power Girl Fitness. powergirlfitness.com. Founded by Jessy Lipke (and her parents) at the age of 10, after seeing her school friends who participated in dance struggle with weight issues and poor self-image. She noticed fitness programs were not available for girls and set out to fill the void.

Power Music. Markets music to the fitness industry. Founded by Richard Petty, who started off mixing custom tapes for instructors-customers.

Powter, Susan. In the 1990s she begged us to "stop the insanity." In 2012, she is out and proud and making web blogs that offer her opinions on a variety of topics related to fitness.

The Putkisto Method. Featured in the article by Jaana Parviainen in *Women and Exercise*. Popular in Europe, the Putkisto Method teaches methods of deep-stretching, deep-strengthening, and deep-breathing. It focuses on muscle tightness as the primary problem in all fitness.

RBG Fit Club. A holistic, healthy lifestyle, and fitness movement founded by hip hop artist Stic (of dead prez). The five core principles of the program are knowledge, nutrition, exercise, rest, and consistency which values pro-active, preventative holistic health.

Rosas, Debbie and Carlos. Creators of the Nia Technique. Carlos retired in 2010, got married, and changed his last name to AyaRosas. Debbie continues to lead trainings and teach classes and her husband, Jeff Stewart, is Nia's CEO.

SharQuí A belly dance fitness brand developed by Oreet, a competitive belly dancer, professional dancer, and fitness instructor. The only fitness-accredited belly dance workout in the world.

Shaun T. (Thompson). Famous for his Hip Hop Abs DVDs as well as for Insanity programs. Also #42 on the Top 100 most influential in 2012.

Shaw, Beth. Creator of YogaFit. Yoga instructor and entrepreneur and president of YogaFit. Her fitness work is also devoted to service, including Shaw's non-profit organization, Visionary Women in Fitness, which provides scholarships to women, and her work as an animal advocate.

Shiva Rea (Trance Dance). Yoga teacher who provides teacher training, retreats, and resources on the holistic nature of yoga (vinyasa).

Silver Sneakers. Created by Healthcare Dimensions, Inc., in 1992. A fitness program specifically designed for senior citizens.

Simmons, Richard. An American fitness personality who promotes weight-loss programs, such as through his *Sweatin' to the Oldies* line of workout videos. He is known for his eccentric personality.

Sorensen, Jacki. Shortly following Cooper's *Aerobics*, Sorensen created dance aerobics.

Stay Human. A yoga apparel company founded by Michael Franti and Carla Swanson. Also connected with Soulshine Bali, a yoga retreat center. A portion of the company's proceeds benefit Bumi Sehat Natural Birthing Clinic in Indonesia and the Hunter's Point Family in San Francisco. Also the name of an album by Franti and Spearhead.

Step (Aerobics). Innovated by Gin Miller after a knee injury in the late 1980s as a lower-impact form of aerobic exercise. An elevated platform, a specially-manufactured "step" (first manufactured by Reebok) is used. While "old-school" step involves a set of moves organized into combinations and routines by individual instructors, BTS and Les Mills have their own versions of step — Group Step and Bodystep, respectively.

32mix.com. A website that provides the fitness community with music, constructed of steady BPM (beats per minute) and 32-count phrases that give energy and momentum.

Title Nine. A clothing line for active women. Named for the legislation that created equal opportunity for girls in sports.

Wai Lana. Fitness television personality (PBS) who also has a line of yoga products including mats, DVDs, and music.

Warner, Jackie. American fitness trainer known for her role on Bravo TV reality show *Work Out.*

Weintraub, Amy. Founder of LifeForce Yoga, senior Kripalu teacher and mentor.

Wii Fit. Video game designed by Nintendo for the Wii gaming console.

Yee, Rodney. Yoga instructor who became popular in the 1990s when he started the series of Gaiam/Living Arts yoga instructional DVDs.

YMCA. A non-profit organization in more than 10,000 communities in the U.S. that provides fitness-related activities and services, with a particular focus on children and community. Established in the 1800s, the YMCA's Christian mission has been downplayed to "the Y ensures that everyone has the opportunity to become healthier, more confident, connected and secure." Diversity and access are important to this organization.

Yoga Ed. A teacher training program aimed to bring yoga into educational settings.

YogaFit. Largest yoga school in the world where instructors train on content to be presented in health club, fitness facilities, and group exercise locations.

Zumba. A trendy fitness program created by Alberto "Beto" Perez. It involves dance and aerobic elements set to Latin music.

Chapter Notes

Intro

1. This is, perhaps, a good place to note two contradictions in my study. First, while I am using this term "American fitness" as a general way of exploring mainstream fitness trends in the United States, this category of "American" is fuzzy. In fact, much of the critical work being done regarding "American" fitness is being done by scholars outside of the U.S. including Canada, Europe, and Australia. American Studies as an academic field has tried to encourage and engage with "American studies" done outside of the U.S., arguing that these outside perspectives shed light in places that American scholars might miss. But this also speaks to the fact that American fitness trends have been cross-pollinated and exported around the world. Second, most of this work is being done from within the social sciences. Even when this work claims, and works to include, interdisciplinary perspectives, the methods, formats, and scope are almost exclusively set within social science parameters. Interdisciplinary scholarship is difficult for a variety of reasons, and part of my work here seeks to illuminate theories and methods toward interdisciplinary research.

2. As Eileen Kennedy and Pirkko Markula explain in their introduction, "Beyond Binaries: Contemporary Approaches to Women and Exercise," their book "takes a tentative step away from binary separations of artificial media image and authentic experience; discourse and embodiment; oppression and resistance; critical feminist researcher and participant in order to create better, transformative fitness practices for women" (16). I also used this idea of binaries in my early work in academia related to fitness: a poster titled "Women's Fitness: Patriarchal Religion or Freedom through Empowerment?" and a presentation about women's work in fitness. The panel: "Reconsidering Women's Work in Global Contexts: From Survival to Activism." My presentation: "Balancing Binaries: The 'Work' of Women's Fitness."

3. The concept of the "Other" comes from postcolonial theory and carries the implication of objectifying or stereotyping a group. The more one group sees another group as "Other," the easier it is to dominate, dismiss, or take advantage of the Othered group. I use this term later when considering issues of cultural appropriation.

Chapter One

1. These fitness definitions can be found on the websites for each of these organizations.

2. Gina Kolata, a science writer for the *New York Times*, explores the idea of fitness through a variety of lenses. In her chapter "History Repeats Itself," Kolata provides a history of fitness that is anchored by Kenneth Cooper's "new fitness movement" and ranges from the Greeks through the eighteenth and early nineteenth century, through the middle of the nineteenth century, the turn of the century, the "golden age of sport" in the 1920s, and the reemergence of fitness

as a national issue after World War II (25–41). This history shows early consciousness and a simplistic, effective approach — a balance. Perhaps it is fitting that the post–World War II fitness fad "began with a call to arms," as Kolata explains. Then it blew up.

3. These height/weight ratio charts are the bane of many women's existence. I reconsider these charts and ratios later in relation to body image and disordered eating.

4. This is a basic premise of feminist critique that has been recognized by a number of scholars and feminist critics. While I simplify these ideas of masculinity as dictum to get bigger and femininity as mandate to get smaller, I am generalizing fitness dictates as well as cultural norms and stereotypes. However, this double standard continues to be a sticking point, a reason why feminism is not obsolete.

5. Kolata (233) and LL Cool J, as well as many others, note this fear. I hear this nearly every day as I pass through fitness spaces, or even at the grocery store or in the halls around my office.

6. For instance, in an "uncategorized" 2008 Wordpress blog post, "CrossFit: Forging elite fitness...at what cost?" an anonymous blogger presents a letter she posted on the CrossFit website. This letter, addressed to "Coach," claimed this blogger as a fan of CrossFit's program while she also pointed out the demeaning ways in which women were portrayed through the CrossFit programs. For instance, using the "motivational" word "pussy" to encourage Cross-Fitters to work harder and the objectification of women through some of the pictures used for promotional purposes. This letter provoked many interesting comments on her site as well as the CrossFit website. Most were defending CrossFit using typical misunderstandings of gender and feminism.

7. While both articles end with an invitation to share "what's on your bucket list," a few days after I saw the article posted there were no comments on the article about the women's bucket list and 101 comments on the men's bucket list. Not surprisingly, many of the comments were questioning the writer's suggestions and credentials. Under-neath the sometimes insulting gendered expectations, some of Murphy's analysis and advice is valuable. In fact, his list for men seems to be far more stereotypical than his list for women, even if his descriptions of women's goals and desires are sexist.

8. This is a common argument in many places. In an article I wrote for *Ethnic Studies Review*, about the TV Show *Survivor*, I discuss the ways in which "better bodies," when defined as young, thin, and tan, are not "better" at all. My studies are rooted in U.S. fitness while making comparative connections outside U.S. borders. What becomes clear, as it is repeated in several variations throughout *Women and Exercise*, is that the ideal of the fit-body, in popular culture and in policy, across countries and westernized cultures, is obsessed with appearance and continually promotes an unattainable ideal. Whether it is age, size, or ethnic or religious tradition, this "ideal" is ultimately a barrier to fitness. Further, the balancing of the demands of cultural and institutional structures with the rewards of lived experiences continue to be illuminated through research about women and exercise even as these are also negotiated through these lived experiences themselves, and are sometimes intertwined.

9. For an excellent discussion of "American ideology," see Howard Zinn's introduction *to Declarations of Independence*. I use this piece in all of my introductory American studies classes.

10. Later I come back to this subject to consider music in another light. Stic Man's 2011 solo album, *The Workout*, carries the themes of "Be Healthy" further, adding new dimensions.

11. *30 Rock* often plays with stereotypes about gender and sexuality. With this example about Michelle Obama, the show is critiquing the ways in which powerful women are portrayed as being manly. Fitness is also fair game on *30 Rock*; Jack's perpetual nemesis, Baines, is a spinning instructor. He comes full of a diva attitude and treats his participants horribly (walking out of class, degrading them). Jack teases Bains about being such a gay stereotype. And Liz is always going to go to the

gym after whatever important task or delicious food item she is committed to.

12. I am particularly perturbed by the fashion of high heels. After developing plantar fasciitis problems when I was teaching 3 classes a day, I began to stick to comfortable shoes. Sensible footwear and yoga and Pilates have mostly healed the problem. So, when I see Beyoncé bouncing around in high heels, modeling this kind of fitness to youth, my feet, and my heart, ache. However, Beyoncé redeemed herself when she demanded that H & M only use "natural" photos of her in their swimsuit campaign. (Dick)

13. I'll note here that several of my students have cited Schwarzenegger's book *The New Encyclopedia of Modern Bodybuilding* as influential to them in the past and present. I don't mention this elsewhere but Arnold continues to be an important figure in American fitness. He regularly posts on the fitness blog on his website schwarzeneg ger.com (which includes a fitness advisory board). Kolata notes that his early influence was, in part, due not simply to his size and strength but also to his movie star celebrity persona, his connections to the Kennedys, and his "engaging" personality. (225) As an inspirational figure in many regards, he is also a controversial figure with a reputation for sexism and misogyny. (Brady 88)

14. The results as told to me by a fitness supervisor. After introducing BTS programming, participation in group fitness classes increased by about fifty percent.

15. Thanks to Amy Stroud for pointing this out to me. I had read this and heard it elsewhere, but I didn't really think about the importance of these aspects. Equal treatment of women in fitness is an important goal toward transformation.

16. All quotes come from the Insanity website. Some are from text but most are from the introductory video.

17. Be Scofield writes about some of the contradictions of yoga being used in the military in "Yoga for War: The Politics of the Divine" (139–140). It is being used to treat PTSD, but we should not assume that yoga is shifting military consciousness toward peace.

18. *Yoga, Inc.* explores how yoga has transformed itself into a commodity and some of the contradictions that arise as a result. It shows the yoga expos, the merchandising, the brands of yoga as well as yoga apparel. A whole subtitled section of the documentary discusses "McYoga," the growth of yoga as a manufactured, branded product. The disagreements, contradictions, competition, commercialization, different/relative "morals" and philosophies, and the tensions between tradition and innovation, spirituality and business are hashed out. One expert proclaims that yoga is an 18 billion dollar business. Yoga sales earn profits, Barry Minkin argues, that are greater than the profits made from the sale of McDonalds,' or Coca Cola, or Gillette in the United States. Such financial stakes mean that mainstream culture is highly invested in fitness.

19. Jaana Parviainen explores the standardized quality of programs like Les Mills in a piece in *European Cultural Studies*, cited in a blog by Pirkko Markula. I make similar arguments here, referring to these types of fitness programs as both "institutionalized" (a part of the bigger structures that contain and shape other leisure and health practices) and "manufactured" (created for the express purpose of wide distribution and profit).

20. Ambivalent feelings and differing tastes are difficult to sort through. While I feel the same way that Markula does about Zumba, other people love — I mean really love — Zumba. In a newsletter produced for a local health and fitness program called Move and Improve, a "featured participant," describes that her "motivation is to keep moving and to inspire others to keep moving." She describes her active past and how she stopped dancing in her 30s. She tried "every 'latest fitness craze'" until she found Zumba and was "immediately addicted." She got certified and now teaches Zumba three times a week. Her answer to what kinds of activities she enjoys is : "Zumba. Zumba and Zumba." Her story is not unique.

21. On May 3, 2005, Tammy and Craig Warman, posted an entry about the split between Les Mills and BTS, which ignited a

conversation on their blog about the similarities and differences. Despite being posted in 2005, the conversation continues to receive comments periodically. Some people see one or the other as better. (Between the two, I prefer BTS for a variety of reasons.) Others wonder what happened to free-style, and lament or curse the rise of manufactured fitness forms like these.

22. Kolata notes that ACSM "takes certification seriously" (245). A bachelor's degree in a health and fitness-related field as well as 900 hours of practical experience is required along with a written and practical test. (245) Thanks also to Danielle Eastman for reminding me about ACSM's more stringent requirements.

23. Stepping into Nia is the concept that begins each class. Stepping out of the daily grind and into a space reserved for movement and joy means being fully present. After class we "step out" more prepared to face our lives.

24. Kolata's source here, Claude Bouchard, notes that there are low responders and high responders and that about 10 percent of the population will show little to no response to training while about 10 percent of the population will respond extremely well to training. (127–131)

25. I first saw this league late one night on MTV. These women can play. But they are forced to play in ridiculous lingerie-like costumes that are only partially obscured by the shoulder pads they wear. The game is spliced and packaged toward entertainment, but the action on the field is a real sporting competition.

26. A much-cited example of the ridiculous standards we have regarding our bodies. See my discussion in *Pictures of Girlhood*, for instance. This aspect of *Mean Girls* is more real than the parodic aspects first reveal; the Plastics exist in many incarnations.

27. Thanks to Danielle Eastman for reminding me that while I may see the silence of Zumba as an emphasis on the body and a distraction from the mind, others may find that the silence of Zumba has the opposite effect. Perhaps a lack of verbal cueing allows participants to focus on their own bodies.

Chapter Two

1. Brabason notes that "body management and surveillance is a reminder of how women — particularly working-class women — are disempowered in post–Fordist economic structures."

2. My focus here, and throughout this book, is on women and on expectations and representations of gender. Certainly there are many dedicated male instructors who exude the qualities I speak to here. In 15 years of teaching, however, I cannot name one I've worked with personally. In so many arenas and so many fitness spaces, specific examples of men's fitness are assumed to include women in the universal sense of humankind. Part of my aim is to provide illustrative examples of American fitness where women's experiences are assumed to be the universal.

3. Academic conventions for citation, and restrictions concerning music copyrights, are difficult to navigate in both academic and fitness spaces. This is a difficult skill to teach students as well, especially as what is public becomes more accessible and adaptable. Shared culture is everywhere.

4. Strober argues that the difficult aspect of "talking across disciplines" is "the way colleagues from different disciplines think — their assumptions; concepts; categories; methods of discerning, evaluating, and reporting 'truth'; and styles of arguing — their disciplinary cultures and habits of mind" (4).

5. For instance, Repko argues that "merely bringing insights from different disciplines together in some way but failing to engage in the hard work of integration is **multidisciplinary studies**, not interdisciplinary studies" (13; original emphasis). See also Strober (16). Interestingly, both Strober and Repko use food metaphors to explain the differences among these terms.

6. Quoting Raewyn W. Connell.

7. Critical studies of race, in and out of academia, are concerned with hair. Hair is contested ground that speaks to issues of femininity, beauty, representation, racism,

white supremacy. For instance, see Chris Rock's documentary, *Good Hair*.

8. I certainly take up these issues as well; they are important for any consideration of gender and fitness in America. One important book that I do not use as a source here is *Critical Bodies: Representations, Practices and Identities of Weight and Body Management*. Edited by Sarah Riley, Maree Burns, Hannah Frith, Sally Wiggins, and Pirkko Markula. This is, in part, due to a lack of access, and part due to my intended purpose. Weight and body management are important aspects of American fitness, and women's fitness in particular, but these concerns are considered here in a wider context, with the emphasis on the ways in which we might transform these concerns in the realm of fitness, if not culture-at-large. Another book that offers a nuanced look at "critical bodies" is Debra Gimlin's 2002, *Body Work: Beauty and Self-Image in American Culture*.

9. I return to the subject of endorphins later. They are a widely noted phenomenon, but little understood. We feel them. As I was finishing this manuscript, the July 2013 Group Groove educational materials arrived at my house from BTS. The campaign (or theme) for this release is "Keep Calm and Groove On." The CD/DVD package cites the Mayo clinic as it describes the effects of endorphins, arguing that exercise helps to improve our mood... and more!

10. In *21st Century Yoga* Remski suggests a service exchange. When you take an hour yoga class and focus on yourself, take another hour to serve others.

11. In using this example I am not suggesting that mainstream limitations to ideas of fitness are in any way comparable to the ways in which black Americans have been limited — violently or structurally — by American culture. However unequal this comparison, the role of the structures of American definitions in the lives of individuals and groups should be explored from as many angles as possible. Double consciousness is a foundational idea to oppositional consciousness and feminist fitness.

12. At a conference a couple of years

later, she passed by me and a colleague doing yoga in the hotel gym on her way to that cardio machine.

13. In *21st Century Yoga* Scofield notes that "spiritual practices can help prevent the burnout associated with activism and social justice work" (134).

Chapter Three

1. In fact, as Kennedy and Markula note, "the responsibility of the healthy looking body is assigned to individual women" (3) by media as much as by personal trainers, for instance. Trainers and instructors also expect us to work hard and look good and to take individual responsibility for doing so. Some research suggests that clients want their trainers and instructors to look "good." (Kennedy and Markula 10)

2. It might be important to note at least two things here. Certainly there can be nothing wrong with wanting to look good, wanting to be feminine, or wanting to wear make-up. However, we should consider what stereotypes of femininity we are trying to live up to and why, and we should consider just *who* we want to look good *for*. Further, when I argue that fitness is not about the outside, but about our health and wellness, I am not ignoring the biological implications that are involved in physical attraction. But it would be misleading to assume that physical attraction on a biological level is about how a person looks. Attraction is certainly based (in part) on how we look on the outside, but the contemporary standards of beauty and body size are not about biology or physiological attraction. These are social constructions and change over time. If physical appearance drove our biological need to attract the opposite sex, men would not be looking for ultra-thin, powdered and pressed, and surgically enhanced; they would be looking for a mate that would protect and care for their young.

3. One of the strengths and weaknesses of feminist research is that the personal is often part of the analysis. This is a strength when considering embodied fitness prac-

tices, and it is also a strength for an understanding of something that can be so personal and yet have larger socio-cultural implications. It is a weakness only in that this work might be discounted by those whose personal, political, or academic beliefs are not informed by feminism.

4. This poem was originally published in the inaugural issue of a local journal: the *Tarratine Quarterly* (issue 1, 2012), along with a piece called "A Feminist Manifesto/a."

5. She notes that Havaron Collins' "study of yoga offers one brave attempt for creating fitness practices informed by feminist principles" (61). If Havaron Collins is the "one brave attempt," then we are not looking in the right places. We are not doing enough to engender feminist fitness.

6. While I have always been interested in "women's issues" and women's studies, I did not start to refer to myself as feminist until I started teaching "Introduction to Women's Studies" in 2009. Teaching this class reinforced for me the importance of using this term despite, or because of, its negative connotations.

7. See, for instance, bell hooks, *Feminism Is for Everybody* or her interview in South End Press's anthology, *Talking About a Revolution*.

8. Part of an interdisciplinary approach means that the practical tools of anatomy and physiology, cueing and execution, could also be complemented by considering philosophy and engagement.

9. Rihanna shows up often in my playlists. Her music is just too perfect for dancing. In the public eye, Rihanna deals with her share of criticism. Such criticism is a pet peeve of mine, particularly the press that she was subjected to after her boyfriend, Chris Brown, hit her and police insiders leaked the photos. While this happened in 2009, it continues to follow her. For an excellent critical analysis of this see Alisa Bierria, "Where Them Bloggers At?" Reflections on Rihanna, Accountability, & Survivor Subjectivity."

10. By "sheltered" I mean being raised by two white, middle class parents (and a television). My parents cared a lot and tried

to compete with the lure of pop culture. I also mean a school career where I was always known as "the smart one" or, in other words, a nerd. I do remember seeing Tupac on *The Cosby Show*, but I did not know who he was or that he had a larger significance outside of his acting and his guest appearance on this show. My love of Hip Hop began in the late 90s, starting when I heard the first few bars of Spearhead's album, *Home*. Similarly, I was too young to know about the Riot Girls but too old to jump on the Spice Girls bandwagon. Thus, my feminist inspirations were mostly through Madonna who pushed the envelope of sexual expression more than any other feminist pursuit. In college, I was introduced to Ani diFranco.

11. I don't remember exactly when I first read this article, but it was sometime around the year 2000. It influenced the work I did regarding fitness in graduate school as I considered her argument about fitness as a "patriarchal religion" but I set this piece aside until I started working on this project and decided to assign it as required reading in my American Fitness class in the fall of 2012.

12. A "Master Class" is an instructional class that is offered to instructors by someone with a lot of expertise in a particular kind of fitness — a "master" trainer. The class often models a certain "brand" of fitness or a particularly innovative approach. These are offered at conferences and expos and are sometimes offered at fitness studios or on college campuses. Depending on place, duration, and popularity, a Master Class might cost at least a hundred dollars, if not more, or it may be free.

13. While I was in the process of writing this book, the information on Alisa Valdes's author's webpage changed dramatically. In 2012, when I looked at her site, it was focused on the promotion of her forthcoming memoir. This book was originally advertised with the title *Learning to Submit: How Feminism Stole My Womanhood, and the Traditional Cowboy Who Helped Me Find It* and was splashed all over Valdes's author's webpage when I was doing re-

search in the fall of 2012. When I went back in 2013, the focus was on her fiction, and there was little mention of the memoir. This new website also includes a "little-known fact" that she is an "AFAA certified group exercise instructor." I speak to some of these changes here as they pertain to Valdes as an illustrative example. The spelling of her name has also changed throughout her career. In *Listen Up* there is an accent mark, and when she got married she hyphenated her name with her husband's name, Rodriguez. Most recently her name is simply spelled as Valdes.

14. Wakeman writes: "instead of writing a story about how she reconciled her feminist views with her desire for a more traditional male partner — a subject which could be useful to many, myself included — Valdes trashes feminism, which strikes me as irresponsible and ungrateful." Critics are generally not sympathetic to Valdes's revelation. One headline from Salon.com sums it up: "The Cowboy Abused the Feminist. What a Surprise."

15. Thanks to Amy Stroud for making this observation. I had not considered that her appearance skirts the edges of child and adult as much as her delivery slips between authority and confidante.

16. Thanks to Ellen Taylor who introduced me to this idea of "kinesthetic" pedagogy. I hadn't considered using this term before she observed my teaching and participated in this class.

17. See Leora Tanenbaum, *Catfight: Women and Competition*. (2002)

18. In fact, in *21st Century Yoga*, Remski describes a kind of "catholic relapse" as he explains the ways in which churches are able to maintain a giving community through outreach programs. (110–12)

19. On the Greatist.com list of "influencers," a significant number have no direct connections to physical fitness. I categorize these "influencers" as "inspirational" figures. These are figures who might promote being happy or balanced, or who might advocate healthy living. They are an eclectic mix of inspirational/motivational personalities (like #10, Dr. Phil McGraw or #20, Tony

Robbins) whose messages can encompass fitness but who might be more connected to mental health than to physical fitness and the (mental) health benefits that can come from physical activity. An intersectional inspirational example comes from journalist Dan Savage (#22) who started "It Gets Better" with his husband, "a project that supports LGBT teens by boosting their self-esteem and offering positive messages from successful adults of all sexual orientations."

20. When I mentioned this site to a yoga friend of mine in Minnesota, a friend who is active in her church, holding a deacon position, and identifying herself as Christian, she reported back to me that she found the site to be a bit "crazy." In fact, I had not intended her to take the site seriously, and she didn't/couldn't. It was way too extreme in its adaptation to be useful to her — both as a fitness instructor/yoga teacher, and as a Christian.

21. Cycling gets less attention as a fitness choice, perhaps because it seems far more complicated. To Gina Kolata, Spinning (a particular brand of indoor cycling) is "serious" (7). It requires specialized equipment which is often expensive, and it requires a mechanical know-how to keep your equipment in working order or to change your tire when you are 20 miles from home and you get a flat. Both running and cycling can be isolated and isolating endeavors as much as communal ones. While cyclists may form themselves into cycling communities and socialize before and after, there is little time for talking when you're balancing on your two wheels — teetering at the edge of the road or speeding down a hill. But cycling also takes place in the studio. In this space, cycling is social and communal. The work of the fitness class requires very little technical know-how and promises a workout that will get your heart pumping and turn your legs to rubber. Movements, and often the cueing as well, emulate the outdoor experience. Some cyclists go into the studio to train; some Spinning participants go outside to ride. Some never cross over.

22. The Wikipedia entry for "Barefoot

Running" is an interesting read for a quick overview of the history and modern phenomenon referred to as "barefoot running" or "natural running." And with specially-designed shoes, it is called "minimalist running."

Chapter Four

1. I can't help but invoke the ghost of Sylvia Plath here. She had many edges in her short life. Her poem "The Mirror" always moves me no matter how many times I have read it. Whenever I think about the mirrors of the studio, and the kind of psychic trauma they produce, I think of the old woman at the bottom of Plath's lake.

2. The extreme case of this obsession with tanning can be seen in the scandalous "tan mom" story. "Tan Mom" made headlines after her children's welfare was called into question because of her tanning practices — not only did she tan, but she had her children tanning as well. Her skin was almost burned black, a frightening sign of her denial. But even when not this extreme, in fitness contexts, tanning is a given. Many studios, and places like 24 Hour Fitness or Snap Fitness, include tanning in their range of services. Bodybuilders tan (quite excessively) in order to better show off their muscles. Even average white women obsess about being "too white" and think they look better with "some color." Too white and some color are certainly culturally weighted concepts.

3. With a little bit deeper searching, one can easily find out that Shaun T is out and proud and married to his partner.

4. Edward Said coined the term Orientalism to describe, in part, the racism of the West in its commodification and exploitation of the Asian "Other."

5. The Power to the Peaceful festival, founded in 2001, was not held in 2011 or 2012, in part because of "rising city fees." (Koskey)

6. In her book, *Shadowboxing*, Joy James writes about segregated and transcendent communities. The yoga community that Franti and others write about can be better understood by a closer look at the ways in which it is a transcendent community. As James argues, "transcendent community is thought to extend through time and space, unbound by spatial or temporal limits; therefore, its 'transcendence' includes the ancestors as well as the present collective and future unborn children. All comprise 'community'" (38).

7. In part Five I return to this subject as I consider race, and specifically, whiteness as the concept and cultural dominance are potentially transformed through fitness.

8. Hot Nude Yoga is illuminated briefly in *Yoga, Inc.,* for instance.

9. It is not entirely coincidental that both of the quotes that begin this chapter are from books about violence against women. Sebold's is a work of fiction, but this fiction draws from the real-life violence she survived, which she writes about in her memoir, *Lucky*. Muscio's work blends her own life experiences with a plethora of information about the "violent times" in which we live. Fitness is one method to combat such violence.

10. For me, part of the fun of a class like Group Groove is being able to try on a masculine stance — to play the man who is in a car full of girls. Besides, I often hear the wrong lyrics. For weeks I thought that Macy Gray was singing about a woman in "Kissed It," until I listened to the original version of the song. Again, that's part of the fun of fitness; you can be yourself, but you can also be a different version of yourself, or someone else entirely.

11. Gay culture/community is certainly present in many gym spaces and (out) gay men are widely accepted as fitness instructors. Jillian Michaels is largely accepted, in part, because she is: attractive, feminine, and a mother. She was also popular before she was out. We could do better to make fitness spaces open and inviting to all people.

12. Octavia Butler is my favorite writer, so I can't help but include at last one reference to her work in everything I write. Here I am specifically referring to Lauren Olamina and her brother, Marcus. Butler writes about these two characters, brother and sister, raised by a "would be world

saver" and each working toward his or her own vision of what the world is and why it might need to be saved. While I quietly considered how I might "save the world" through my contributions to a variety of larger, radical causes, Erin saw herself as working to "save the earth." Her concern was not with people, but with the planet.

13. *Feminist Pedagogy*, Introduction (5): "Feminist teaching uses an ethic of care (Gilligan 1982); some have even used the word *love* (see, for example, hooks [1994, 1995, 1996], who explores the erotic nature of teaching, and Wallace's [1999] psychoanalysis of practicing feminist pedagogy)."

14. The editors/authors of the Introduction to *Feminist Pedagogy* note the influences of Paulo Freire's use of the term liberatory pedagogy (2000), and feminist critique of this work as well as that of Freire's "disciples": Henry Giroux (1997), Peter McLaren (2000), and Ira Shor (1996). While I read some of Freire's work in graduate school and was familiar with some of Giroux's work, I was formally unaware of this work on pedagogy, no doubt absorbing these ideas from an education provided by professors familiar with this work.

15. A summary of what Krista Scott-Dixon explains in her article "Big Girls Don't Cry: Fitness, Fatness, and the Production of Feminist Knowledge."

16. See Anna Clark's "The Foodie Indictment of Feminism" on Salon.com. May 26, 2010 and *The New York Review of Books*, "The Food Movement Rising" by Michael Pollan, June 10, 2010.

17. It is also important to note here that Johnson's blog was posted in 2010 and had two years to attract comments before Game's blog. And yet, when I stumbled upon these conversations, Game's was the post that had been given the most cyber-attention.

18. From Michael Kimmel, "A Black Woman Took My Job." He writes about the four pillars of masculinity: No Sissy Stuff, Be a Big Wheel, Be a Sturdy Oak, and Give 'Em Hell.

19. A different kind of "bell curve" might argue that LL Cool J's "god-given genetics" are inferior to genetics of other "races." However, race is a social construct, not a biological reality. There is no gene or set of genes that are shared by all members of the same "race." See the PBS series *Race: The Power of an Illusion* for the basics. From there it's much more complicated, mostly because the vast majority of Americans misunderstand what "race" really is.

20. By mundane, I suppose I mean the "universal" struggles of humankind that are distilled in the worries of the middle/upper classes. For instance, having babies and dealing with parents' divorce. She also describes the "striving" involved in her "unsustainable cultural obsession with having the best" (202). As she insists on an exclusive private school education since public school is somehow not good enough for her daughter, Dederer reflects that "this striving was entirely reflected in my yoga" (203). To be fair, the events Dederer shares are, perhaps, no more mundane than the aspects of my life that I choose to share here. The mundane is an important site for transformation.

Chapter Five

1. Many authors discuss the current prison system as a version of slave labor. For instance, consider Joy James, *Shadowboxing*, where she points out that the Thirteenth Amendment does not end slavery but makes it legal as a condition of imprisonment. Or, see Angela Davis, *Are Prisons Obsolete?*

2. bell hooks uses this term across her many works. In an October 2012 talk at Colby College in Waterville, ME, she adds "imperialist" to the list.

3. The adaptable Revolutionary But Gangsta (RBG) acronym (also red, black, and green) is morphed into Reaching Bigger Goals on the RBG store site. This shift might seem to undercut the revolutionary message of "revolutionary but gangsta," but perhaps it also speaks to flexibility. An acronym can have multiple meanings.

4. It's important to note at least two things here. First, Bruce Lee and Joe Louis both fought racism in their own ways and both provide positive heroes and role models for young boys, particularly boys of

color. Second, there are the occasional references to female heroes like Jackie Joyner in "Runner's High."

5. See for instance, greatveganathletes. com as well as the June 20, 2012 *NY Times* article by Gretchen Reynolds, "Can Athletes Perform Well on a Vegan Diet?"

6. YogaFit, for instance, directly intervenes through YogaLean and an emphasis on "mindful eating."

7. In using this example I am not suggesting that mainstream limitations to ideas of fitness are in any way comparable to the ways in which black Americans have been limited — violently or structurally — by American culture. However unequal this comparison, the role of the structures of American definitions in the lives of individuals and groups should be explored from as many angles as possible. Double consciousness is a foundational idea to oppositional consciousness.

8. Michael Stone explores the possibilities of the 99 percent in his piece in *21st Century Yoga*. Essentially he reads the Occupy movement(s) as a starting point for "collectively imagining the future" (160). While he makes many important points here, the "mind" part of mind/body fitness might be overrated. He writes, "being able to change our mind *is* enlightenment. Maybe being able to change the structures within and around us is the activation of our deepest, hard-won insights" (160; original emphasis).

9. I had previously participated in a Zumbathon with a handful of other instructors and had enjoyed it. We used a microphone and we practiced ahead of time and shared the stage the whole time. Many elements were the same; both events had a rotation of instructors, a stage, special outfits, door prizes, a large crowd. But this Zumbathon was a different experience.

10. Lugones makes the distinction between male-dominated Western "play," which is really just competition, and feminist, "'world'-travelling" play. In a keynote address at our University of Maine at Augusta 2013 English Student Conference, Ruth Ozeki, described the relationship between writer and reader, or text and reader,

as a dynamic like play. She had begun to describe it like a game and then corrected herself to say it is not quite a game, but like play.

11. Dill and Zambrana explain that intersectional analysis "is characterized by the following four theoretical interventions": "(1) Placing the lived experiences and struggles of people of color and other marginalized groups as a starting point for the development of theory; (2) Exploring the complexities not only of individual identities but also group identity....; (3) Unveiling the ways interconnected domains of power organize and structure inequality and oppression; and (4) Promoting social justice and social change by linking research and practice to create a holistic approach ..." (5). The tenants speak to feminist mind/body fitness through an emphasis on lived experience, group identity, structured inequalities, and linking research and practice.

12. From onebillionrising.org. The site cites the 2003 UNIFEM report entitled "*Not a Minute More: Ending Violence Against Women,*" or 2008, the *UNITE to End Violence Against Women Campaign*, initiated by UN Secretary-General's Office as the sources for this statistic.

13. Remski also offers a list for both practitioners and studio owners that lists "what we can do" (124–6). I don't offer similar lists here; they are embedded, embellished, and in progress.

14. This principle is explained in part by: "The Japanese have the wisdom to promote pleasure as one of their goals of healthy living. In our fury to be thin and healthy, we often overlook one of the most basic gifts of existence — the pleasure and satisfaction that can be found in the eating experience."

15. Patanjali is credited with compiling the yoga sutras, a set of ideas that form what we know as yoga. This book is considered the most important and influential to an understanding of the eight-limbs of yoga, and it is used for a variety of types of yoga. Patanjali is not credited with inventing yoga, but with bringing together knowledge from a variety of sources and many yogis have offered a variety of commentaries on the text.

Works Cited

Writing a book that brings together a variety of sources from academic books and articles, to personal blogs, to internet stories, to televisions shows and music, to personal experiences and local examples, makes a works cited section particularly difficult to compile and navigate. I have opted to list all of my cited resources — books, DVDs, articles, websites — in one section rather than separate them according to type of publication. Chapters from books have been listed individually by the last name of the author since this is how I cite them in the text. When an author is available, websites are listed by the author's name; otherwise, they are listed by the name of the website.

I also have not included the dates I accessed the websites cited here. Most of the research and writing for this book was done 2012-2013. All sites were accessed during 2012-2013. Several websites changed during this time, Alisa Valdes's official website was renovated and her blog through blogspot.com was removed (which I discuss in detail in "My Generation and Beyond"), RBG Fit Club was upgraded in 2013, and YogaFit's website was also upgraded in 2013. The description for Feminist Figure Girl also changed while I was in the process of writing this book.

Sources that are only listed as suggestions or references in my endnotes are not listed here, unless I quote from these sources or these sources are also quoted in the text of the book. Sources that are mentioned but not quoted from are also not listed here. Further descriptions of fitness terms, products, brands, and personalities can be found in the appendix.

Allen-Collinson, Jacquelyn. "Running Embodiment, Power and Vulnerability: Notes Toward a Feminist Phenomenology of Female Running." *Women and Exercise: The Body, Health, and Consumerism.* Pirkko Markula and Eileen Kennedy, Eds. Routledge Research in Sport, Culture and Society. United Kingdom: Routledge, 2010. 280-298. eBook.

Al-Rawi, Rosina-Fawzia. *Grandmother's Secrets: The Ancient Rituals and Healing Power of Belly Dancing.* Translated by Monique Arav. New York: Interlink Books, 2003. Print.

American Psychological Association. "Sexualization of Girls Is Linked to Common Mental Health Problems in Girls and Women-Eating Disorders, Low Self-Esteem, and Depression; An APA Task Force Reports." 19 Feb. 2007. Web.

Arkin, Daniel. "Zumba Instructor Sentenced to 10 Months in Jail on Prostitution Charges." NBC.com. 31 May 2013. Web.

Bass, Clarence. "*Aerobics* Marks 40-Year Anniversary." Ripped Enterprises. *cbass.com.* 2008. Web.

Beachbody. *Beachbody.com.* 2013. Web.

Bechdel, Alison. *The Essential Dykes to Watch Out For.* New York: Houghton Mifflin Harcourt, 2008. Print.

bell hooks: Cultural Criticism and Transformation. Dir. Sut Jhally. 1997. Video.

Belli, Giocanda. *The Country Under My Skin: A Memoir of Love and War.* New York: Anchor Books, 2003. Print.

Bendrix, Trish. "Susan Powter Thinks It Should Be Obvious She's a Lesbian." *AfterEllen.com.* 11 Nov. 2008. Web.

Bennett, Bija. *Emotional Yoga: How the Body Can Heal the Mind.* New York: Fireside (Simon & Schuster), 2002. Print.

Billups, Andrea. "Jason Russell 'Healing' After KONY 2012 Video Led to Naked Street Rant."*People.com.* 8 Oct. 2012. Web.

Boynton, Victoria. "Women's Yoga." *My Life at the Gym: Feminist Perspectives on Community Through the Body.* Jo Malin, ed. New York: SUNY Press, 2010. Print.

Brabazon, Tara. "Fitness Is a Feminist Issue." *Australian Feminist Studies.* 21.49 (2006): 65-83. Web.

Brady, Jacqueline. "Beyond the Lone Images of the Superhuman Strongwoman and Well-Built Bombshell Toward a New Communal Vision of Muscular Women." *My Life at the Gym: Feminist Perspectives on Community Through the Body.* Jo Malin, ed. New York: SUNY Press, 2010. 79-90. Print.

Broad, William J. *The Science of Yoga: The Risks and Rewards.* New York: Simon & Schuster, 2012. Print.

Brown, Christina. *The Yoga Bible: The Definitive Guide to Yoga Postures.* Cincinnati, OH: Walking Stick Press, 2003. Print.

Caitlin. "Fit and Feminist." Fitandfeminist. blogspot.com. Web.

Carrellas, Barbara. "Welcome to Barbara Carrellas.com and Urban Tantra.org (asm)!" *BarabaraCarrellas.com.* n.d. Web.

Carroll, Linda. "Toned Teens: Most Teen Boys and Girls Trying to Build Muscles." Vitals on *NBC News.com.* 9 November 2012. Web.

Clark, Tena. "Break the Chain." *OneBillionRising.org.* 2013. Web.

Cooper, Kenneth. *Aerobics.* New York: Bantam Books, 1968. Print.

Cooper Aerobics Health and Wellness. Cooper Aerobics. 2013. Web.

Coulter, Myrl. "Gym Interrupted." from *My Life at the Gym: Feminist Perspectives on Community Through the Body.* Jo Malin, ed. New York: SUNY Press, 2010. 101-109. Print.

Couples Retreat. Dir. Peter Billingsley. Perf. Vince Vaughn, Jason Bateman. Universal Pictures, 2009. DVD.

Crabtree, Robin D., David Alan Sapp, Adela C. Licona, eds. "Introduction: The Passion and Praxis of Feminist Pedagogy." *Feminist Pedagogy: Looking Back to Move Forward.* Baltimore: Johns Hopkins University Press, 2009. Print.

"CrossFit: Forging Elite Fitness ... at What Cost?" *wordpress.com.* 10 May 2008. Blog.

Dederer, Claire. *Poser: My Life in Twenty-three Yoga Poses.* New York: Farrar, Straus, and Giroux, 2011. Print.

Dick, Emily Lauren. "Average Girl." *Loveaverage.com.* Web.

_____. "H&M Following Suit and Changing Their Ways." Average Girl. Loveaverage.com. 31 May 2013. Web.

Dill, Bonnie Thornton, and Ruth Enid Zambrana, Eds. *Emerging Intersections: Race, Class, and Gender in Theory, Policy, and Practice.* New Brunswick, New Jersey: Rutgers University Press, 2009. Print.

Douglas, Susan J. *The Rise of Enlightened Sexism: How Pop Culture Took Us from Girl Power to Girls Gone Wild.* New York: St. Martin's Grifin, 2010. Print.

DuBois, W.E.B. "Of Our Spiritual Strivings." *The Souls of Black Folk.* New York: Dover Publications, 1994 (1903). Print.

Durrett, April. "Dance-Inspired Classes Big in Venezuela." World Beat column. October 2010. *IDEA Fitness Journal.* 96. Print.

_____. "Taking Exercise Al Fresco in Spain." World Beat Column. July-Aug. 2010 *IDEA Fitness Journal*. 128. Print.

East Bay Express. "Reader's Poll Winners: Sports and Leisure." Eastbayexpress.com. 2012. Web.

Easton, Dossie, and Catherine A. Liszt. *The Ethical Slut: A Guide to Infinite Sexual Possibilities*. Eugene: Greenery Press, 1997. Print.

Eltham, Ben. "The Copyright Cops." *Inside Story: Current Affairs and Culture from Australia and Beyond*. 15 July 2010. Web.

Emery, Debbie. "What Caused Madonna's Scary Arms?: New Pictures of the Material Mom Reveal That No Matter How Much You Exercise, You Can't Fool Father Time." *Betty Confidential*. 30 Jul. 2009. Web.

Enlighten Up! Dir. Kate Churchill. Perf. B.K.S. Iyengar, Pattabhi Jois. DOCU-RAMA, 2009. DVD.

Feminist Fitness. *Feministfitness.tumblr.com*. n.d. Web.

Franti, Michael and Carla Swanson. "Stay Human: Apparel, Yoga, Gear." StayHumanNow.org. Web.

Friel, Brianne. "An Interdisciplinary Introduction to Women's Studies." New York: Gival Press, LLC, 2005. Print.

Game, Kevin Smith. "Feminism is Making America Fat." Château Heartíste. 28 June 2012. Blog.

Girls on the Run. 2013. Web.

The Greatest Team. "The 100 Most Influential People in Health and Fitness 2012." 20 Dec. 2012. *Greatist.com*. Web.

Groven, Karen Synne and Kari Nyheim Solbrække and Gunn Engelsrud. "Large Women's Experiences of Exercise." *Women and Exercise: The Body, Health, and Consumerism*. Pirkko Markula and Eileen Kennedy, Eds. Routledge Research in Sport, Culture and Society. United Kingdom: Routledge, 2010. 121-137. eBook.

Healthy Is the New Skinny. n.d. Web.

Hentges, Sarah. *Pictures of Girlhood: Modern Female Adolescence on Film*. McFarland, 2006. Print.

Hipline.myhipline.com. 2011. Web.

hooks, bell. *Feminism Is for Everybody: Passionate Politics*. Cambridge: South End Press, South End Press. 2000. Print.

_____. *Teaching Community: A Pedagogy of Hope*. New York: Routledge, 2003. Print.

_____. *Teaching to Transgress: Education as the Practice of Freedom*. New York: Routledge, 1994. Print.

_____, and Amalia Mesa-Bains. *Homegrown: Engaged Cultural Criticism*. Cambridge, MA: South End Press, 2006. Print.

Hollywood Homicide. Dir. Ron Shelton. Perf. Harrison Ford, Josh Hartnett, Lena Olin. Sony Pictures Home Entertainment, 2003. DVD.

Horton, Carol. *Introduction: Yoga and North American Culture. 21st Century Yoga: Culture, Politics, and Practice*. Carol Horton and Roseanne Harvey, eds. Chicago: Kleio Books, 2012. Print.

Houser, Catherine. "Enduring Images." *My Life at the Gym: Feminist Perspectives on Community Through the Body*. Jo Malin, ed. New York: SUNY Press, 2010. 91-93. Print.

Insanity. Beachbody.com. 2013. Web.

Intuitive Eating. "10 Principles of Intuitive Eating." 2013. Web.

James, Joy. *Shadowboxing: Representations of Black Feminist Politics*. New York: Palgrave (St. Martin's Press), 1999. Print.

Jensen, Marlene. "Walking Is an Exercise in Friendship." *My Life at the Gym: Feminist Perspectives on Community Through the Body*. Jo Malin, ed. New York: SUNY Press, 2010. 151-154. Print.

Johnson, Janet Elise. "Beyond the Burn: Toward a Feminist Fitness." *Bitch Magazine*. 2006. Print.

Johnson, Lisa. "Feminism Makes You Fat." Lisa Johnson Fitness. 28 May 2010. Web.

Keira. Fit Feminist. *Fitfeminist.blogspot.com*. n.d. Web.

Kell, Tiffany. "Project Bendypants: Practicing Yoga While Fat." *Decolonizing Yoga*. n.d. *More Cabaret*. 3 Apr. 2013. Web.

Killen, Rob. "Fitness and Churches-A Growing Trend." *Faith and Fitness Magazine*. n.d. Web.

Kimmel, Michael. "A Black Woman Took

My Job." *New Internationalists*. 373 (2004): n. page. Web.

King of the Hill. "Hank's Back." Season 8, Episode 20. FOX. Aired May 9, 2004. TV.

Klein, Melanie. "How Yoga Makes You Pretty: The Beauty Myth, Yoga and Me." *21st Century Yoga: Culture, Politics, and Practice*. Carol Horton and Roseanne Harvey, eds. Chicago: Kleio Books, 2012. Print.

Kolata, Gina. *Ultimate Fitness: The Quest for Truth About Exercise and Health*. New York: Picador/Farrar, Straus and Giroux, 2003. Print.

Koskey, Andrea. "Power to the Peaceful Falls Silent for a Second Year." *Sfexaminer.com*. 9 Aug. 2012. Web.

Lattuca, Lisa R. *Creating Interdisciplinarity: Interdisciplinary Research and Teaching among College and University Faculty*. Nashville: Vanderbilt University Press, 2001. Print.

Let's Move! America's Move to Raise a Healthier Generation of Kids. *letsmove. gov*. n.d. Web.

LL Cool J (James Todd Smith) and Dave Honig with Jeff O'Connell. *LL Cool J's Platinum Workout*. New York: Rodale, 2007. Print.

Lokman, Paula. "Becoming Aware of Gendered Embodiment: Female Beginners Learning Aikido." *Women and Exercise: The Body, Health, and Consumerism*. Pirkko Markula and Eileen Kennedy, Eds. Routledge Research in Sport, Culture and Society. United Kingdom: Routledge, 2010. 266-279. eBook.

Lopez, Erica. *The Girl Must Die: A Monster Girl Memoir*. New York: Monster Girl Media, 2010. Print.

Lorde, Audre. *Sister Outsider*. New York: Crossing Press, 2007. Print.

Lugones, María. "Playfulness, 'World'-Travelling, and Loving Perception." *Making Face, Making Soul/Haciendo Caras: Creative and Critical Perspectives by Women of Color*. Gloria Anzaldua, ed. SanFancisco: Aunt Lute Books, 1987. Print.

Malin, Jo. "Introduction." *My Life at the Gym: Feminist Perspectives on Community Through the Body*. Jo Malin, ed. New York: SUNY Press, 2010. 1-15. Print.

Mansbridge, Jane. "The Making of Oppositional Consciousness." *Oppositional Consciousness: The Subjective Roots of Social Protest*. Jane Mansbridge and Aldon Morris, eds. Chicago: U of Chicago P, 2001. Print.

Mansfield, Louise. "Fit, Fat and Feminine? The Stigmatization of Fat Women in Fitness Gyms." *Women and Exercise: The Body, Health, and Consumerism*. Pirkko Markula and Eileen Kennedy, Eds. Routledge Research in Sport, Culture and Society. United Kingdom: Routledge, 2010. 81-100. eBook.

Markula, Pirkko. "Feeling Guilty About Faking Joy." Fit Femininity. *Psychology Today*. 6 February 2013. Web.

_____. "'Folding': A Feminist Intervention in Mindful Fitness." *Women and Exercise: The Body, Health, and Consumerism*. Pirkko Markula and Eileen Kennedy, Eds. Routledge Research in Sport, Culture and Society. United Kingdom: Routledge, 2010. -60-78. eBook.

_____. "It's Fun When It's Over." Fit Femininity. *Psychology Today*. 14 May 2012. Web.

_____, and Eileen Kennedy. "Introduction: Beyond Binaries: Contemporary Approaches to Women and Exercise." *Women and Exercise: The Body, Health, and Consumerism*. Pirkko Markula and Eileen Kennedy, Eds. Routledge Research in Sport, Culture and Society. United Kingdom: Routledge, 2010. 1-25. eBook.

Marsh, Sophie. "The Power of Love-One Billion Rising." *NiaNow.com*. 1 Mar. 2013. Web.

McCall, Timothy, M.D. *Yoga as Medicine: The Yogic Prescription for Health and Healing*. A *Yoga Journal* Book. New York: Bantam, 2007. Print.

McTavish, Lianne. Feminist Figure Girl: Look Hot While You Fight the Patriarchy. *Feministfiguregirl.com*. n.d. Web.

McWilliams, Jenna. "Susan Powter Is a Lesbian." *Jennamcwilliams*. Making Edible Playdough Is Hegemonic: Notes Toward Resistance. 12 July 2012. Web.

MC Yogi. *Elephant Power.* Velour Recordings, 2008. CD.

MC Yogi. *Pilgrimage.* Velour Recordings, 2012. CD.

"Meet the Man Behind Zumba: Beto Perez." *Reader's Digest.* Nov. 2009. Web.

Meyer, Heather Alaine. *Create Your Own Beautiful.* 2012. Web.

Miss Representation. 2011. Web.

Moraga, Cherrie, and Gloria Anzaldua. *This Bridge Called My Back: Writings by Radical Women of Color.* New York: Kitchen Table, 1984. Print.

Morris, Aldon and Naomi Braine. "Social Movements and Oppositional Consciousness." *Oppositional Consciousness: The Subjective Roots of Social Protest.* Jane Mansbridge and Aldon Morris, eds. Chicago: University of Chicago Press, 2001. Print.

"Move and Improve." Volume 10, Issue 1. March 3-March 9, 2013. e-Newsletter.

Murphy, Laura. "Seventeen agrees to promote realistic beauty." *Worldoncampus. com.* 10 July 2012. Web.

Murphy, Myatt. "Fitness Bucket List for Guys." Innovation for Endurance. *MSN.Fitbie.* 20 Aug. 2012. Web.

_____. "Fitness Bucket List for Women." Innovation for Endurance. *MSN.Fitbie.* 20 Aug. 2012. Web.

Muscio, Inga. *Rose: Love in Violent Times.* New York: Seven Stories Press, 2010. Print.

National Women's Studies Association. n.d. Web.

Newhall, Kristine. "You Spin Me Right Round, Baby." *My Life at the Gym: Feminist Perspectives on Community Through the Body.* Jo Malin, ed. New York: SUNY Press, 2010. Print.

Nordqvist, Joseph. "African American Women Avoid Exercise Because of Hair Maintenance." *Medical News Today.* 19 Dec. 2012. Web.

Oliver, Chyann L. "for sepia 'colored girls' who have considered self/when hip-hop is enuf." *Home Girls Make Some Noise: Hip Hop Feminism Anthology.* Aisha Durham, Gwendolyn D. Pough, Rachel Raimist, and Elaine Richardson, eds. Mira Loma, CA: Parker Publishing, LLC., 2007. Print.

Pabon, Jorge. "Popmaster Fabel." *Physical Graffiti: The History of Hip Hop Dance.* *Total Chaos: The Art and Aesthetics of Hip-Hop.* Jeff Chang, Ed. New York: Basic Civitas Books, 2007. 18-26. Print.

Park, Roberta J., "Prologue: Reaffirming Mary Wollstonecraft! Extending the Dialog on Women, Sport and Physical Activities." In *Women, Sport, Society: Further Reflections, Reaffirming Mary Wollstonecraft.* Eds. Roberta J. Park and Patricia Vertinsky. Sport in the Global Society series. New York: Routledge, 2011. Originally published in the *International Journal of the History of Sport,* vol. 27, issue 7. Print.

_____. "Women as Leaders: What Women Have Attained in and Through the Field of Physical Education." In *Women, Sport, Society: Further Reflections, Reaffirming Mary Wollstonecraft.* Eds. Roberta J. Park and Patricia Vertinsky. Sport in the Global Society series. New York: Routledge, 2011. Print.

Parker-Pope. "Go Easy on Yourself, A New Wave of Research Urges." *New York Times.* 28 Feb. 2011. Web.

Parks and Recreation. "Live Ammo." Season 4, Episode 19. NBC. Aired April 19, 2012. TV.

Parviainen, Jaana. "Women Developing and Branding Fitness Products on the Global Market: The Method Putkisto Case." *Women and Exercise: The Body, Health, and Consumerism.* Pirkko Markula and Eileen Kennedy, Eds. Routledge Research in Sport, Culture and Society. United Kingdom: Routledge, 2010. 44-59. eBook.

"Patricia Krentcil Case: Tanning Mom Trial Sent to New Jersey Grand Jury." *Huffingtonpost.com.* 4 June 2012. Web.

Petersson McIntyre, Magdalena. "Keep Your Clothes On! Fit and Sexy Through Striptease Aerobics." In *Women and Exercise: The Body, Health, and Consumerism.* Pirkko Markula and Eileen Kennedy, Eds. Routledge Research in Sport, Culture and Society. United Kingdom: Routledge, 2010. eBook.

Pharr, Suzanne. "Homophobia: A Weapon

of Sexism." *Women's Voices, Feminist Visions: Classic and Contemporary Readings.* Susan M. Shaw and Janet Lee, eds. New York; McGraw-Hill, 2012. 5th ed. 71-74. Print.

Pike, Elizabeth C. J. "Growing Old (Dis)Gracefully? The Gender/Aging/Exercise Nexus." *Women and Exercise: The Body, Health, and Consumerism.* Pirkko Markula and Eileen Kennedy, Eds. Routledge Research in Sport, Culture and Society. United Kingdom: Routledge, 2010. 180-196. eBook.

Power Girl Fitness. *Powergirlfitness.com.* 2011. Web.

Powter, Susan. *Susanpoweter.com.* n.d. Web.

Price, Catherine. "Weight Loss: How Women Do the Math." *O Magazine.* Oprah.com. July 2008. Web.

Pugh, Christina. "An Elegy for Dancing." *My Life at the Gym: Feminist Perspectives on Community Through the Body.* Jo Malin, ed. New York: SUNY Press, 2010. 19-30. Print.

PUP. Perfectly Unperfected Program/Project. *Healthy Is the New Skinny.* 2011. Web.

RBG Fit Club. Raising the Bar. Upgrade Season 2013. *rbgfitclub.com.* 2013. Web.

Remski, Matthew. "Modern Yoga Will Not Form a Real Culture Until Every Studio Can Also Double As a Soup Kitchen, and Other Observations from the Threshold Between Yoga and Activism." *21st Century Yoga: Culture, Politics, and Practice.* Carol Horton and Roseanne Harvey, eds. Chicago: Kleio Books, 2012. Print.

Repko, Allen F. *Interdisciplinary Research: Process and Theory.* Los Angeles: SAGE press, 2008. Print.

Restaurant Impossible. "Mr. Irvine Goes to Washington." Season 3, Episode 13. Food Network. Aired June 13, 2012. TV.

Rich, Emma and John Evans and Laura De Pian. "Obesity, Body Pedagogies and Young Women's Engagement with Exercise." *Women and Exercise: The Body, Health, and Consumerism.* Pirkko Markula and Eileen Kennedy, Eds. Routledge Research in Sport, Culture and Society. United Kingdom: Routledge, 2010. 138-157. eBook.

Richter, Amy, Rev. "The Ripped, Bikini-Clad Reverend." *The New York Times Magazine.* 20 Apr. 2012. Web.

Roff, Chelsea. "Starved for Connection: Healing Anorexia Through Yoga." *21st Century Yoga: Culture, Politics, and Practice.* Carol Horton and Roseanne Harvey, eds. Chicago: Kleio Books, 2012. Print.

Rosas, Debbie and Carlos. *The Nia Technique: The High-Powered Energizing Workout That Gives You a New Body and New Life.* New York: Broadway Books, 2004. Print.

Rosman, Katherine. "Group Fitness Classes Use Music to Compete for Clients: Zumba to 'Ice Ice Baby'" *Wall Street Journal.* Home & Digital, 6 Feb 6, 2013. Web.

Roth, Gabrielle. *Connections: The Five Threads of Intuitive Wisdom.* New York: Jeremy P. Tarcher/Penguin, 2004. Print.

Rushkoff, Douglas. *The GenX Reader.* New York: Ballantine Books, 1994. Print.

Sandoval, Chela. *The Methodology of the Oppressed.* Theory Out of Bounds. Minneapolis, London: University of Minnesota Press, 2000. Print.

Schlosser, Eric. *Fast Food Nation: The Dark Side of the All-American Meal.* New York: Perennial, 2002. Print.

Schultz, Jaime. "The Physical Is Political: Women's Suffrage, Pilgrim Hikes and the Public Sphere." *Women, Sport, Society: Further Reflections, Reaffirming Mary Wollstonecraft.* Eds. Roberta J. Park and Patricia Vertinsky. Sport in the Global Society series. New York: Routledge, 2011. Print.

Scofield, Be. "Yoga for War: The Politics of the Divine." *21st Century Yoga: Culture, Politics, and Practice.* Carol Horton and Roseanne Harvey, eds. Chicago: Kleio Books, 2012. Print.

Scott-Dixon, Krista. "Big Girls Don't Cry: Fitness, Fatness, and the Production of Feminist Knowledge." *Sociology of Sport Journal.* 25.1 (2008): 22-47. Print.

Shaw, Beth. *Beth Shaw's YogaFit.* Second Edition. Champaign, Illinois: Human Kinetics, 2009. Print.

Siddha Yoga. "Ashram in Oakland: Prison Project." *Siddhayoga.org.* 2012. Web.

Simmons, Richard. "A Biography of Richard Simmons." RichardSimmons.com. n.d. Web.

Simpon, Andrea. "Why Gaga Believes In Yoga's Higher Healing Power." *Celebuzz. com.* 4 Apr. 2013. Web.

Speak Out! Biography and Booking Information. "Ericka Huggins: Human Rights Activist, Poet and Scholar." *Speakoutnow. org.* Web.

Stic Man. *The Workout.* BOSS UP, INC, 2011. CD.

Stoeffel, Kat. "The Feminist and the Cowboy Author Leaves Abusive Cowboy." The Cut. *NY Style.com.*11 Jan. 2013. Web.

Stone, Michael. "Our True Nature Is Our Imagination: Yoga and Non-Violence at the Edge of the World." *21st Century Yoga: Culture, Politics, and Practice.* Carol Horton and Roseanne Harvey, eds. Chicago: Kleio Books, 2012. Print.

Strober, Myra H. *Interdisciplinary Conversations: Challenging Habits of Thought.* Stanford: Stanford University Press, 2012. Print.

Stump, Scott. "'Kony 2012' Filmmaker on Public Meltdown: 'I Was Not in Control of My Mind.'" *News Today.* 12 Oct. 2012. Web.

Tavakoli, Shaden. "This DJ." *Home Girls Make Some Noise: Hip Hop Feminism Anthology.* Aisha Durham, Gwendolyn D. Pough, Rachel Raimist, and Elaine Richardson, eds. Mira Loma, CA: Parker Publishing, LLC., 2007. Print.

Thealogian. Fat Feminist Fitness Blog. *FatFeministFitnessBlog.blogspot.com.* 1 Aug. 2011. Web.

30 Rock. "Unwindulax." Season 7, episode 4. NBC. October 25, 2012. TV.

Valdés, Alisa. "How the Body Reminds the Spirit What Matters." *Buena Vida.* 2 Apr. 2013. Web.

_____. "Learning to Submit: Questioning Extreme Feminism's Impact on Romance, Love, and Relationships." alisavaldesrodriguez.blogspot.com. 2012.Web.

_____."Ruminations of a Feminist Fitness Instructor." *Listen Up: Feminist Voices from the Next Generation.* Portland; Seal Press. 2001. Print.

Verbrugge, Martha H. "Recreation and Racial Politics in the Young Women's Christian Association of the United States, 1920s-1950s." *The International Journal of the History of Sport.* 27.7 (2010): 1191-1218. Print.

Vogel, Amanda. "Generation X: From Slackers to Stars, the Future of Fitness." *Idea Fitness Journal.* July 2011. Print.

Wachob, Jason. "Robert Downey Jr. Gets His Yoga On." *Mind.Body.Green.* 15 Jan. 2012. Web.

Wade, Megan. "Feminist Fitness Books." *Feministing.com.* 26 Sept. 2009.

Wakeman, Jessica. "On Alisa Valdés' Conflict with Feminism, Her Cowboy & Domestic Abuse." *thefrisky.com.* January 14, 2013. Web.

Walter-Bailey, Wendy. "If These Roads Could Talk: Life as a Woman on the Run." *My Life at the Gym: Feminist Perspectives on Community Through the Body.* Jo Malin, ed. New York: SUNY Press, 2010. 145-149. Print.

Warren, Frank. *Post Secret.* n.d. Web.

Weaver, Jane. "Can Stress Actually Be Good for You?" *msnbc.com.* 20 Dec. 2006. Web.

Weintraub, Amy. "LifeForce Yoga." *Yogafor depression.com.* 2013. Web.

Wescombe, Libby. "Oh Fitness Industry, Where Art Thou Balance?" *Eatercise blog.* 4 Nov. 2012. Web.

Wharton, James C. *Crusaders for Fitness: The History of American Health Reformers.* New Jersey: Princeton University Press, 1982. Print.

Wielebinski, Grace. "'Skinny Girls Don't Have Oomph!': Vintage Weight Gain Ads." *BUST Magazine.* Style File. 25 July 2012. Web.

Williams, Alexandra. "Kazakhstan: A Rich Cultural History with Fit New Ideas." World Beat column. *IDEA Fitness Journal.* Sept. 2010. 104. Print.

_____. "Thailand: An Ancient-Modern Fitness Marriage." World Beat column. *IDEA Fitness Journal.* Nov.–Dec. 2010. 96. Print.

Willis, Laurette. "Why a Christian ALTERNATIVE to Yoga?" *Praise Moves.* 2007. Web.

Woodard, Marcia. "The Gymnastics Group." from *My Life at the Gym: Feminist Perspectives on Community Through the Body*. Jo Malin, ed. New York: SUNY Press, 2010. 95-100. Print.

Wray, Sharon. "The Significance of Western Health Promotion Discourse for Older Women from Diverse Ethnic Backgrounds." *Women and Exercise: The Body, Health, and Consumerism*. Pirkko Markula and Eileen Kennedy, Eds. Routledge Research in Sport, Culture and Society. United Kingdom: Routledge, 2010. 161-179. eBook.

Y.O.G.A. for Youth. "Our Mission." *Yogaforyouth.org*. n.d. Web.

Yoga, Inc. Dir. John Philp. Perf John Abbott, Baron Bapitste, Jimmy Barkan. Bad Dog Tales, 2007. DVD.

Yoga Is: A Transformational Journey. Dir. Suzanne Bryant. Perf. Russell Simons, Christy Turlington-Burns. Magnolia Home Entertainment, 2012. DVD.

The Yoga Sutras of Patanjali, Translation and Commentary by Sri Swami Satchidananda. Originally published as: *Integral Yoga: The Yoga Sutras of Patanjali*. Yogaville, Virginia: Integral Yoga Publications, (1978) 2007. Print.

Young, Susan. "From Ballet to Boxing: The Evolution of a Female Athlete." *My Life at the Gym: Feminist Perspectives on Community Through the Body*. Jo Malin, ed. New York: SUNY Press, 2010. Print.

Index